PRAISE FOR

Postpartum Depression Demystified

"In this clear, comprehensive, easy-to-read book, Venis and McCloskey take their readers step by step through recognizing and deciding what they need to do to recover from postpartum disorders. Their personal and professional experience allows them to know and understand the subject and communicate it in a caring, sensitive way. Recommended for moms and health providers. We need more books like this!"

—DIANE G. SANFORD, PHD,
*Women's Health Expert for the American Psychological Association
and Coauthor of* The Postpartum Survival Guide

"Sophisticated in content, yet highly readable, *Postpartum Depression Demystified* is destined to become a classic, must read choice for mothers, families, and practitioners alike when seeking an informative, comprehensive, and compassionate resource on pregnancy related mood disorders. Emphasizing the treatable nature of these illnesses, *Postpartum Depression Demystified* offers a hopeful path to recovery through its attention to the importance of community connections and comprehensive guide of available treatment options. Venis and McCloskey draw upon their immeasurable experience and decades of clinical expertise to present an authoritative resource that meets the challenge of this mental health crisis with intelligence and sensitivity."

—SUSAN DOWD STONE, MSW, LCSW,
*President, Postpartum Support International,
NJHSS Certified Perinatal Mood Disorders Instructor*

"Every new mom and family member should have a copy of *Postpartum Depression Demystified*. This book explains, in a simple form, what every mom should know. I wish this book had been written five years ago."

—CAROL BLOCKER, *whose daughter suffered from postpartum psychosis*

"As a health-care professional in the maternal and child health field, I see *Postpartum Depression Demystified* as a thorough, interesting, and informative source of education—not just for those who suffer from PPD, but also for their partners and families—while also serving as a validation for those who are symptomatic of this disorder. The format is easy to read and it also can be utilized as a reference for health-care professionals when identifying women with PPD. This book is a most timely must read for both professionals and the general public."

—CATHERINE VIEIRA, CARN, CPAS, CCE

JOYCE A. VENIS, RNC, is a psychiatric registered nurse and the past president of Depression After Delivery, Inc., which has recently merged with Postpartum Support International. With more than thirty years of experience, she is nationally recognized for her work and expertise in the subjects of perinatal mood disorders, premenstrual syndrome (PMS), perimenopause, and menopause. A PPD survivor herself, she is the founder and director of the Princeton Pregnancy and Postpartum Support Group. Venis lectures extensively, has appeared on a number of television and radio shows, and has been interviewed for various publications, including *Newsweek,* the *Chicago Sun, Parenting,* and *Parents.* She has been asked to testify before Congress, participated in the formulation of a state resolution, and was an instrumental witness for a PPD case in New Jersey. In 2005 Governor Cody appointed Venis to the New Jersey PPD Task Force, where she helped significantly increase PPD awareness throughout the state. She lives in central New Jersey.

SUZANNE McCLOSKEY is a former Marlowe & Company editor, where she acquired and edited many books on health, psychology, relationships, and parenting, including, in the Demystified series, *Borderline Personality Disorder Demystified.* She lives with her family in Westchester County, New York.

Postpartum

Depression

Demystified

Postpartum Depression Demystified

AN ESSENTIAL GUIDE TO UNDERSTANDING AND
OVERCOMING THE MOST COMMON COMPLICATION
AFTER CHILDBIRTH

Joyce A. Venis, RNC,
and Suzanne McCloskey

MARLOWE & COMPANY ■ NEW YORK

POSTPARTUM DEPRESSION DEMYSTIFIED: *An Essential Guide to Understanding and Overcoming the Most Common Complication after Childbirth*

Published by
Marlowe and Company
An imprint of Avalon Publishing Group, Incorporated
245 West 17th Street • 11th Floor
New York, NY 10011-5300

The information in this book is intended to help readers make informed decisions about their health and the health of their loved ones. It is not intended to be a substitute for treatment by or the advice and care of a professional health-care provider. While the authors and publisher have endeavored to ensure that the information presented is accurate and up-to-date, they shall not be held responsible for loss or damage of any nature suffered as a result of reliance on any of this book's contents or any errors or omissions herein.

Library of Congress Cataloging-in-Publication Data

Venis, Joyce A.
    Postpartum depression demystified : an essential guide to understanding and overcoming the most common complication after childbirth / Joyce A. Venis, and Suzanne McCloskey.
      p. cm.
    Includes bibliographical references and index.
    ISBN-13: 978-1-56924-266-7 (trade pbk.)
    ISBN-10: 1-56924-266-6 (trade pbk.)
    1. Postpartum depression. 2. Puerperal psychoses. I. McCloskey, Suzanne.
II. Title.
RG852.V46 2007
618.7'6—dc22

                                                                    2006039024

9 8 7 6 5 4 3 2 1

Designed by Pauline Neuwirth, Neuwirth & Associates, Inc.

Printed in the United States of America

For Chris and Jack—SM

∞

For Mark, Malcolm, and my patients—JV

CONTENTS

There are times in every life when we feel hurt or alone . . .
But I believe that these times when we feel lost
and all around us seems to be falling apart are really bridges
of growth.
We struggle and try to recapture the security of what was,
But almost in spite of ourselves, we emerge on the other side
with a new understanding, a new awareness, a new strength.
It is almost as though we must go through the pain
and the struggle
in order to grow and reach new heights.
—Sue Mitchell

INTRODUCTION

MOST WOMEN NEVER expect to have postpartum depression. They spend their pregnancies full of nervous and joyful anticipation, preparing for their baby's arrival and dreaming of the future. They read all the usual books and take the recommended childbirth education class, none of which address postpartum depression in anything more than a trivial way. They know from movies, television, books, and magazines that having a baby will be the most joyous and wonderful experience of their lives, and that they will feel only happiness, satisfaction, and pride after the baby is born. Why should they imagine it would be any other way?

Unfortunately, close to seven hundred thousand new moms *do* develop postpartum depression every year, and the majority of them are completely unprepared for the fallout. A large part of the blame for this must be placed on our society's attitude toward motherhood. Our culture has been very reluctant to talk about the reality of having a baby and the enormous physical, emotional, and relationship changes that it brings. In fact, society seems intent on perpetuating antiquated, unrealistic expectations of new mothers that should have disappeared long ago. We are bombarded with images of new moms happily baking cookies and cleaning the house while their husbands are at work and then contentedly rocking their babies to sleep at night (and, of course, the baby is never crying), which has created an impossible standard for us to try to meet. When our babies are born,

we are expected to know exactly what to do and how to do it, even though we've had no training or instruction. If we have a C-section or a difficult birth, we shouldn't be upset or traumatized; we should just feel grateful that we have a baby. We are expected to return, unchanged, to our old selves immediately after childbirth, even though our hormones are fluctuating wildly and we have just embarked on a radical life change. When we don't conform to the cookie-cutter expectations society has for its new mothers, we are judged harshly. There is something wrong with us if we're not happy. Not only are these expectations unrealistic; they're also damaging. Our culture has actually helped perpetuate postpartum depression, because it has made women afraid and ashamed to admit they are having problems after their babies are born and to seek help when they need it.

Here's the reality: the days, weeks, and months after childbirth can be overwhelmingly difficult, and having a baby marks the beginning of one of the biggest life changes you will ever go through. You're recovering from the physical trauma of giving birth, your hormones have gone haywire, you're sleep deprived, and now you are completely responsible for every aspect of another human life. You'll have to reevaluate and reprioritize your relationships with everyone in your life, because caring for your baby has to come first now. You feel overwhelmed and unsure of yourself much of the time. Life with baby is not the way you imagined it would be, and you may feel disappointed, sad, and angry about that. You may feel guilty because you're not happy and therefore not living up to people's expectations. And that's just the tip of the iceberg. There are dozens of other biological, psychological, and social risk factors that make you more susceptible to postpartum depression. Is it any wonder that up to 20 percent of new mothers develop the condition every year?

Society's views on mental health issues, particularly those related to motherhood, have also added to the stigma attached to postpartum depression. Our culture tends to reject people with mental health issues, believing they should be able to "snap out of it" on their own, which is impossible. People don't talk about postpartum depression, which means the public at large doesn't understand what it is. Society continues to use poor examples to illustrate postpartum depression—for instance, many people believe that Andrea Yates, the woman who drowned her five kids in the bathtub in June 2001, had postpartum depression when she actually suffered from postpartum psychosis, a much rarer and far more severe postpartum mood disorder. All of this works to further discourage women from talking about their feelings and seeking help, because they are afraid of being stereotyped as "crazy." They are far from crazy and suffer from a true medical illness.

What Can We Do to Change Things?

In order to make the postpartum period easier for mothers and make help for postpartum depression more accessible, we need to adopt a new view of motherhood that is based in reality. Being a mother is tremendously rewarding, but it is also full of challenges and difficulties. Parenting is hard work; in fact, it is the hardest job on earth. It's not always fun or immediately gratifying. There is no rule book for us to consult to make sure we're doing things right. It's impossible to avoid making mistakes now and then. It's actually very common for women to have all sorts of negative feelings in the weeks and months following childbirth. Society needs to accept the good and the bad aspects of motherhood and stop placing impossibly high expectations on new mothers. On the flip side, new mothers also need to stop placing impossibly high expectations on themselves.

We need to stop looking up to the celebrity moms who lose all of their baby weight in one month and look happier and more fabulous than ever. Unlike most of us, they have personal trainers, cooks, and all day long to dedicate to getting back into shape. And chances are they are not as happy as they look.

People also need to understand that postpartum depression is a real and treatable medical illness, not a mental defect or a character flaw. Having postpartum depression should be no more embarrassing than having diabetes. Our culture should be just as accepting of women with PPD as we are of those with diabetes.

The public needs to be better informed about postpartum depression, and we need to start talking about it more openly. Hundreds of thousands of women suffer from this common and treatable illness every year, but not enough people know that. Postpartum depression should be discussed in every obstetrician's office, every childbirth education class, and among mothers and their families everywhere. This will help women feel more secure about admitting they are having trouble after childbirth and seeking out the proper resources to help them recover.

Why We Wrote This Book

There are several reasons why we thought writing this book was important. First, we have both been through postpartum depression and understand firsthand how desperate and hopeless women with PPD can feel. If you've picked up this book because you have—or suspect you have—postpartum depression, it's important for you to know that you are not alone, that you are not crazy, that help is available, and that you *will* get better. We have two very different tales of postpartum depression, which we share below to offer you some measure of comfort and show you that PPD can strike absolutely anyone.

Joyce's Story

Joyce got pregnant at the age of nineteen in the late 1960s. Despite dropping out of nursing school, marrying the baby's father in a "shotgun wedding," and having an array of other PPD risk factors, Joyce felt great during her pregnancy. She wanted her baby more than anything and abortion was never an option, but after the birth Joyce plummeted into depths of despair—she cried all night long and **intrusive thoughts** constantly plagued her. She went to twenty-two different health-care practitioners seeking help over a long period of time, and many of them wanted to have her hospitalized. They told her she felt this way because she was nineteen and married to someone who didn't want to be married. No one ever told her she had postpartum depression, or even mentioned the term to her. She finally sought psychiatric help because she couldn't sleep. The psychiatrist prescribed fifteen sleeping pills at a time for her, and Joyce saved forty-five pills for a suicide plan. She had decided that over-dosing was going to be the way she would end her pain and that her son would be better off without her. However, a close friend and the psychiatrist Joyce was seeing intervened, and with their help, Joyce eventually worked through her PPD. Once she was better, she real-ized that there was a reason for all of the pain she went through. She had found her calling. Joyce went back to nursing school and became certified in psychiatry, hoping to help other women through their struggles with postpartum depression and other perinatal mood dis-orders. Joyce has spent the last thirty years doing just that, through individual counseling, leading support groups (she started the first PMS support group in New Jersey), and working with postpartum depression organizations like Depression After Delivery, of which she was president for many years. She appreciates her experience with PPD because she feels she is a better person for it and can empathize with her patients. As she likes to tell them, "No one can truly under-stand unless they've been there."

Sue's Story

When Sue found out she was pregnant, she decided she wanted to do things as "naturally" as possible. She chose a midwife, took the childbirth education classes, and prepared for a pain-medication-free childbirth. Her pregnancy went well, with no complications. When her due date came and went, her midwife suggested she try several different herbal remedies to encourage labor to begin. Nothing worked. Finally, nine days overdue, Sue drank castor oil (it was unspeakably horrible), and her water broke an hour later. Her labor went slowly, and when she arrived at the hospital the next morning, she was only two centimeters dilated. The hours dragged on, but she still wasn't dilating. Her midwife suggested an epidural, thinking it might help Sue relax and dilate. Sue agreed, and five hours later she was ready to push.

After an hour and a half of pushing, the baby's heart rate began to drop, and Sue's midwife decided the baby was too big and she needed a C-section (turns out he was eleven pounds). Sue had to wait another hour and a half with no pain medication, struggling not to push with each contraction, until the midwife was ready to deliver her baby. It was excruciating, and when she cried for something to help stop the pain, her midwife bent down and said, "Do you know you haven't even asked how your baby is doing? Why don't you concentrate on him for a while?" The C-section itself was a terrible experience as well. Sue was completely unprepared for everything that had happened. She hadn't given much thought to a C-section, because she was sure she'd give birth naturally. Nothing went the way it was supposed to. She had terrible trouble breast-feeding and had to bring her three-week-old son to the hospital because he had lost a pound. She felt exhausted, overwhelmed, inadequate, and helpless. She cried all the time, over any little thing. She worried about going back to work three months before she had to. She worried about finding the right child care, and most of all about having to find someone else to take care of her baby. She felt she had made a huge mistake having a baby, and wished she could have her old life back. She went on like this for five months until she started having debilitating panic attacks, which finally drove her to seek help. It wasn't until then that she even knew she had postpartum depression. None of her friends had ever talked about feeling this way—she felt alone and thought something must be wrong with her. She decided to find out as much as she could about the condition by reading books and doing research. She realized that there was an urgent need for accessible information on PPD, and she wanted to help other women who were going through what she went through. She read about Joyce on the Depression After Delivery Web site and called her to see if she might like to collaborate on a book. *Postpartum Depression Demystified* is that book.

Another key reason we wrote this book is that we believe it is vitally important to get the word out on postpartum depression and try to help educate women and the public about this condition. We've written this book to make it easier for you to understand what you are going through and to find the support and resources you need to recover. We want to encourage you to take a positive attitude toward the adversity that you feel, to advocate for yourself, and to help change society's perception of this medical problem. Far too many women and families have suffered and continue to suffer because they are afraid or embarrassed to get help, or they don't even know that they have postpartum depression, because they don't understand what it is. Our hope is that *Postpartum Depression Demystified* will empower women and their families to speak out when they are suffering and ask for help. It may not seem so now, but you *will* be better and stronger for this experience.

Who This Book Is For

First and foremost, we wrote this book for women who are suffering from postpartum depression to provide education, comfort, and validation. This book will also be very useful and informative for the partners, children, extended family, and friends of women with PPD. We offer some specific advice to help them cope with their loved one's condition. *Postpartum Depression Demystified* was also written with health-care practitioners in mind, because they need to understand postpartum depression from their patients' perspective in order to provide the best possible care.

How This Book Can Help You

Postpartum Depression Demystified provides accessible, in-depth information on PPD that will help you become an informed and active participant in your health and happiness. You'll learn about the risk factors for postpartum depression; the symptoms; how it's diagnosed; which health-care professionals you should see; what you can do to take care of yourself; how to get the support you need from your partner, family, and friends; and much more. In addition, we offer easy-to-follow tips and advice that will help you ease your symptoms and overcome this illness, as well as quotes from other women who have been there. We also include advice for your partner, family, and friends on how they can best support you through this difficult time. Terms that appear in **boldface** indicate that they are defined in the glossary on page 213. Please note that this book should be used in conjunction with (and not in place of) a health-care practitioner's medical care, and you should always keep your health-care team informed of everything you're doing to help overcome PPD.

A Note about the Term "Partner"

We'd like to make it clear that while we refer to your partner as "he" throughout the book, we do so only for the sake of clarity and convenience. All of the information and advice we provide for the partners of women with PPD is applicable for both men and women partners.

ONE

What Is Postpartum Depression?

MANY OF US have heard the term "postpartum depression" before but don't know exactly what it means. Unfortunately, there is no easy answer to this question. Postpartum depression (also referred to as PPD) is a serious mood disorder experienced by some women after giving birth. It affects approximately 20 percent of new mothers and is considered the most common complication of childbirth. Postpartum depression is generally defined as *a state of persistent sadness or anxiety that lasts longer than two weeks after giving birth,* but the truth is that it's far more complex than that. It can start during pregnancy (as **antepartum depression**) and may continue on after you give birth. It can happen to women after an abortion, miscarriage, **interrupted pregnancy**, or a stillbirth. It can strike women who had easy pregnancies and deliveries and no history of emotional problems or depression. Women who adopt babies have developed PPD, and some women experience it months and even years after giving birth or when they wean their babies. The symptoms vary with each individual and appear in differing degrees. Postpartum depression can last for several weeks, or if left untreated or treated improperly, it can linger on for two years or more. In other words, postpartum depression is a different experience for everyone. This makes the condition more difficult to recognize and therefore treat, both for the women living with it and for their physicians.

The Symptoms

There is a wide range of PPD symptoms that women can experience, but the most common are sadness, anxiety or panic attacks, feelings of hopelessness and guilt, insomnia, and thoughts of harming the baby or oneself (see chapter 2 for a detailed discussion of PPD symptoms). The symptoms can appear within days of giving birth, or they can creep up on you slowly and not become evident for weeks or even months after your baby is born. In fact, PPD can occur anytime within the first year after you give birth. There are even cases of women developing postpartum depression two years after childbirth when they wean their babies. Such was the case for Hyla F., who had a smooth postpartum period and happily nursed her daughter Morgan for two years. When she stopped nursing, postpartum depression hit her hard, and she felt like her world just "fell apart."

As we mentioned earlier, PPD symptoms and their severity are unique to every woman, but in every case postpartum depression is a debilitating condition—it affects your ability to function normally and take care of your child to some degree, and it won't disappear on its own as the more typical baby blues do. (See page 13 for more information on the baby blues.) You must seek treatment from a health-care practitioner, and therapy and medication are usually necessary to help you recover from it.

What Causes PPD?

There is no single explanation for why women develop postpartum depression. For a long time, experts believed it was strictly a biological response to giving birth—a reaction to the craziness of our hormones returning from pregnancy to pre-pregnancy levels. But now we know that adoptive mothers, grandmothers, and even fathers can all experience PPD and that many birth mothers, who also have hormonal changes, do not develop the condition. These factors have led many researchers to believe that the causes of postpartum depression are psychological and sociological as well as biological. Research has also found that women with a history of depression face a greater risk of developing PPD, as do women who were depressed during their pregnancies. Those who suffered PPD after one birth are more likely to develop the condition with subsequent ones. The bottom line is that postpartum depression occurs in different women for different reasons.

Biological Factors

Childbirth is a natural event, but it's also a traumatic event for your body. Unlike menstruation, which your body goes through 400 to 450 times in your lifetime, you give birth only a handful of times. Any woman who has experienced **premenstrual syndrome (PMS)** knows how influential the fluctuation of hormones can be on your mood and feelings of well-being. Think about how nine months of hormonal fluctuations could affect you. When you're pregnant, your body goes through enormous physical changes in which its natural equilibrium is turned upside down, and then it experiences the biggest change of all—birth. During pregnancy, the female reproductive hormones **estrogen** and **progesterone** increase ten times. Within three days of delivery, those levels drop to those of pre-pregnancy. The hormone **prolactin**, which is necessary for milk production, is low after birth but increases dramatically in the first week postpartum to accommodate breast-feeding. The placenta stimulates the production of **endorphins**, which stimulate a feeling of well-being while you're pregnant. After you give birth, your endorphin levels drop abruptly. While scientists have not proven it conclusively, these hormonal shifts are believed to play a role in the development of postpartum depression.

Psychological Factors

When you're sleep-deprived and overwhelmed with the job of caring for your newborn, minor problems can seem much bigger. It's not unusual for women to have a difficult time coping with things that they considered easily manageable before they had their babies, and this can lead to frustration, depression, and anxiety. Other emotional influences that may contribute to postpartum depression include:

- a difficult delivery, especially a Caesarean birth
- an unsatisfying birth experience, such as having your partner called away or having medical complications that make it difficult to care for your baby
- a lost sense of identity—of who you were before your baby was born
- having anxiety, doubts, or unrealistic expectations about being a good mother or having the perfect baby
- excessive weight gain
- feeling less attractive
- feeling disappointed with the baby's gender

Social Factors

The postpartum period is a time of great upheaval in your life, whether this is your first child or your fourth. Studies show that the quality of your relationships, particularly your relationship with your partner, and the support you receive from your family and friends has a big influence on whether you develop postpartum depression. It's very important to have a good relationship with your partner and strong social support system (see chapter 3 for more information on risk factors). Here are some other social conditions that can contribute to PPD:

- young or old first-time mothers
- single mothers
- a baby with a high level of needs, such as colic
- exhaustion from caring for a new baby or multiple children
- pressure to breast-feed
- financial problems
- postpartum pain or delivery complications

- problems with breast-feeding
- low socioeconomic status
- a recent move
- unrealistic expectations of you from others ("She's just a little baby . . . how hard can it be?")

Postpartum Depression Is Different from the Baby Blues

Many women (and some health-care practitioners as well) don't understand the differences between postpartum depression and the "baby blues," and this is a huge reason why so many women with PPD don't seek help or are misdiagnosed. "Baby blues" is the term used to describe the highs and lows that the majority of women go through in the first two weeks or so after giving birth. Having the baby blues is a normal biological reaction to childbirth, and it ends on its own rather quickly (see page 14 for a more detailed discussion of the baby blues). Postpartum depression and the baby blues share many of the same symptoms, but they are two distinct conditions. When you have the baby blues, symptoms like weepiness and anxiety come and go and are interspersed with periods of happiness and contentedness. In contrast, there is little or no relief from the negative symptoms of postpartum depression. It is a far more serious condition than the baby blues—the symptoms are more debilitating, they last a lot longer, they will not go away on their own, and they must be treated by a physician.

To add to the confusion between these two conditions, sometimes PPD begins as a case of the baby blues. If the "normal" baby blues symptoms you're experiencing last longer than three weeks, get worse instead of going away, or more serious symptoms like intrusive thoughts surface, you may have postpartum depression.

Other Perinatal Mood Disorders

Postpartum depression is often used as a blanket term to describe any negative emotional reaction a woman has after childbirth, but it's really only one of several kinds of **perinatal mood disorders** that women can experience. While the focus of this book is on postpartum depression, it's important for you to know the facts about all the different kinds of perinatal reactions so that you're better able to distinguish PPD from the rest.

Antepartum Depression

Antepartum depression, or depression during pregnancy, is extremely common—in fact, studies show that it may be even more common than postpartum depression. Many women who are depressed during pregnancy go undiagnosed because they assume their symptoms are a normal part of pregnancy. Some of the symptoms, such as fatigue and trouble sleeping, are common for healthy women during pregnancy, but when they're accompanied by a sense of sadness or hopelessness and interfere with your ability to function for longer than two weeks, antepartum depression is most likely to blame.

About half of the women who are depressed during their pregnancy will go on to develop postpartum depression, so early detection and treatment of antepartum depression are critical. Both psychotherapy and antidepressant medication are used to treat the condition, and proper treatment will reduce your chances of developing postpartum depression. Another reason why treating antepartum depression is so important is that studies show that if left untreated, it can pose a serious risk to the baby. Untreated depression can lead to poor nutrition, drinking, smoking, and suicidal behavior, which can then lead to premature birth, low birth weight, and developmental problems in the baby. A woman who is depressed often does not have the strength or desire to adequately care for herself or her developing baby, which is why problems arise.

The Baby Blues

Some women appear to breeze through their postpartum adjustment period—they feel wonderful, happy, and confident in their ability to take care of their new babies. But most women—about 85 percent of us—experience what's commonly referred to as the "baby blues," or a mix of negative feelings after giving birth. Symptoms of the baby blues include irritability, rapid mood swings, tearfulness, and anxiety, and they usually begin about two days after childbirth. The baby blues are considered a "normal" postpartum reaction because they are relatively mild and last about two weeks, or as long as it takes for your hormones to settle. Once your hormones are settled, the blues disappear and you feel like yourself again. An important factor in distinguishing the baby blues from PPD or any other type of perinatal mood disorder is that the baby blues do not interfere with everyday functioning. You are still fully capable of taking good care of yourself and your baby. The baby blues also resolves itself quickly and on its own. No medication or therapy is required.

Postpartum Adjustment Disorder

Postpartum adjustment disorder (PPAD) is a condition where women feel anxiety, self-doubt, tearfulness, fatigue, and many of the symptoms of the baby blues, except it lasts for their first two months postpartum instead of just two weeks. Approximately one in five women suffer from postpartum adjustment disorder, but most are never diagnosed or ask for help, because the symptoms are not as severe as postpartum depression. In some ways PPAD is a "normal" part of adjusting to life as a new mother, even though it feels far from normal when you're going through it. Becoming a parent is considered a life crisis from a developmental perspective, and a certain amount of stress and negative feelings after childbirth are considered normal. Most women do go through some variation of postpartum adjustment disorder. Women with PPAD function quite well, but feelings of disappointment and unhappiness and the pressures of being a good mother interfere with their ability to enjoy their babies and feel good about themselves.

> *"I had no idea how I got to this place. It was extremely difficult to adjust to my new life, and I yearned for my old life and freedom. I did not want to baby-proof my*

home. I did not want to give up my ability to shower or even go to the bathroom when I had to."

—Sheri R.

Postpartum adjustment disorder is very treatable with therapy and support groups. Since the symptoms are milder than in postpartum depression, medication is not generally used.

Postpartum Mania

Postpartum mania is primarily triggered by hormonal changes following childbirth. Women with postpartum mania feel "speeded up" and find it difficult to slow down and relax. They often have less of a need for sleep, sleeping maybe two or three hours a night and not feeling tired. Women with postpartum mania give the impression that they must "get it all said and done." Their normal thinking patterns tend to become an uncontrollable rapid flow from one topic to another (racing thoughts), and their speech patterns reflect this, making it difficult for listeners to follow them at times. A woman with postpartum mania is like a ball of energy, making list upon list of things that need to be accomplished, excessively cleaning her house, or taking on difficult projects. But she's so wound up, scattered, and disorganized that she jumps from task to task without finishing them and leaves a mess in her wake.

> *"I could not stop talking or cleaning. I could not sleep, relax, or just stop myself even for a moment. I insisted that what I was doing was important and had to be done, even scrubbing the bathroom floor at 3 AM. I was set in fast-forward."*
>
> —Kerry B.

We usually think of mania as a happy or euphoric mood, but that's not the case with postpartum mania. Women with this condition are mainly just highly irritable and excitable. In the whirlwind of having a baby and adjusting to life after you come home, it's easy to miss the signs of postpartum mania, but the symptoms will quickly build to the point where they interfere with your ability to take care of yourself and your baby. Mania is successfully treated with medication and therapy.

Postpartum Anxiety and/or Panic Disorder

Learning to care for a child can be quite stressful, and feelings of anxiety are not uncommon. But women who are affected by a **postpartum anxiety and/or panic disorder** experience excessive and often irrational worries and fears about their babies as well as their own actions. For instance, a woman with postpartum anxiety and/or panic disorder may constantly worry that she is underfeeding or overfeeding her baby. She may also be plagued with what we call the "what ifs." A woman who has the "what ifs" will worry about what might happen if she doesn't hear her baby cry during the night, or what might happen if she's not stimulating her baby enough. These types of excessive worries can lead to debilitating panic attacks, which are terrifying and can strike at any time and without warning. Many women feel especially nervous, agitated, apprehensive, and tense because they fear another attack. (It's important to note that having just one panic attack does not mean you suffer from postpartum anxiety and/or panic disorder.) They also may experience overwhelming anxiety, and possibly even **agoraphobia**.

> "I had to leave the cart in the grocery store and get out. There was too much going on around me. The lights were too bright, and there were too many decisions that I couldn't seem to make. Should I get the peas or the carrots? I was afraid I was going to lose it in the store, and that sent me into a panic."
>
> —Laura P.

Experts aren't sure exactly why postpartum anxiety and/or panic disorder occurs in some women. Some believe this condition is caused by the additional activity in the **noradrenergic** and **serotenergic**

systems in the brain. This leads to greater **neurotransmitter** activity, which can act as a trigger for panic attacks. Others argue that some women just have a genetic predisposition to developing the disorder. Another theory is that anxiety may be learned behavior, which develops into something more consuming when a person is placed under great stress. Regardless of its source, postpartum anxiety and/or panic disorder can be successfully treated.

Postpartum anxiety and/or panic disorder usually occurs within the first few days after birth, but it can also appear more gradually during the first year after birth. Women with this disorder can suffer from a wide variety of symptoms, including:

- fear of losing control
- feelings of wanting to run away
- feeling anxious about having anxiety
- difficulty relaxing
- insomnia (not due to the baby)
- believing that others can see that they are anxious or in a panic
- feelings of extreme uneasiness for prolonged periods of time
- emotional eating
- jumbled thoughts
- difficulty concentrating
- feeling like they are "jumping out of their skin"
- physical symptoms such as chest pain, rapid breathing, shakiness, and dizziness

Women who have a past history of anxiety or panic attacks are more likely to develop the postpartum disorder. Additionally, those with a family history of anxiety and/or panic disorders have an increased risk of developing postpartum anxiety and/or panic disorder.

Women who are diagnosed with this disorder are typically treated with antianxiety drugs or antidepressants, such as Paxil, and anxiolytics, such as Xanax, Ativan, and Klonopin, which are taken only when needed. Psychotherapy and support groups are also part of the treatment, and in some cases, therapy alone may be enough to help a woman get over this disorder.

Postpartum Obsessive-Compulsive Disorder (PPOCD)

Obsessive-compulsive disorder (OCD) is a condition in which a person becomes consumed with particular thoughts, impulses, or images. These thoughts or impulses cause a great deal of anxiety, disgust, guilt, and discomfort, and as a result, people with OCD have compulsive urges that help them ease their feelings of anxiety and distress.

The difference between **postpartum obsessive-compulsive disorder** and the obsessive-compulsive disorder that affects the general population is that women with PPOCD usually focus their obsessive thoughts on their baby. While women with this disorder may be susceptible to bizarre thoughts, they are intensely aware of the fact that their feelings are not normal. However, some women with PPOCD are reluctant to seek help, because they are afraid they will be looked down upon for their peculiar thoughts and fears.

> *"I kept a chart of when the baby pooped, how much the baby pooped, the color, and the consistency. I just felt I had to do it, over and above anything else. No one was allowed to change the baby but me. They may have missed one."*
>
> —Jess R.

Typical symptoms of PPOCD are disruptive to a woman's daily routine and usually get in the way of her personal relationships. The rituals that many women establish to cope and deal with their obsessive thoughts can be time-consuming and can interfere with regular activities. Signs of postpartum obsessive-compulsive disorder include:

- intrusive, recurrent, and obsessive thoughts, usually involving the baby

- avoidance behavior, possibly of the baby but generally of anything that causes them fear
- establishing rituals that include repetitive behavior, obsessive cleaning or washing, and hoarding objects
- anxiety or depression

Women who are affected by PPOCD usually experience obsessive thoughts about their baby being harmed. This can result in repetitive behavior such as repeatedly sterilizing the baby's bottle for fear that it may be contaminated or checking on the child an excessive number of times. Some women may also harbor fears that they will harm their child in some way, such as drowning the child during bath time. These fears can be especially disturbing, but very few mothers with PPOCD are likely to actually harm their child in any way.

Although any woman has the potential to develop PPOCD, women who have a personal or family history of obsessive-compulsive disorder have an increased risk of developing the condition. Women who develop an obsessive-compulsive disorder during their pregnancy are more than two times as likely to have PPOCD.

There are different treatment options available to women with PPOCD. Therapy is the most effective and valuable way to cope with and change the thoughts and behaviors that accompany PPOCD. Some women may also be treated with anti-obsession and SSRI medications (see chapter 5 for an in-depth discussion on SSRI medications). With proper care and treatment, it is possible for a woman to overcome this disorder.

Postpartum Post-Traumatic Stress Disorder

When we think of **post-traumatic stress disorder (PTSD)**, usually we think of a war veteran who has witnessed unspeakable acts, or catastrophic events like September 11. But there are instances where the act of giving birth is so traumatic that it causes the mother to suffer from post-traumatic stress disorder. The emotional trauma of having to undergo an emergency C-section, having anesthesia ineffectively delivered during a C-section (causing the woman to feel pain during the procedure), having a difficult vaginal birth, and losing your child during the birth can all trigger postpartum PTSD.

Women who are suffering from **postpartum post-traumatic stress disorder** can experience many of the traditional symptoms of PTSD, such as flashbacks and nightmares about the trauma and emotional numbness, but the most common symptom is panic attacks. Postpartum PTSD often strikes women who experienced a loss of identity and control during their deliveries, and are wracked with a sense of loss over the situation.

Postpartum PTSD is treated with medications and therapy.

Postpartum Psychosis

Postpartum psychosis (PPP) is the most severe form of postpartum mood disorder, and also the most uncommon. It occurs in one or two out of every one thousand births, and it usually begins in the first forty-eight to seventy-two hours after childbirth, though it can occur even up to six weeks afterward. Postpartum psychosis symptoms usually appear suddenly and can include delusions, hallucinations, paranoia, bizarre thoughts, religious ideations, and severe agitation. While women with postpartum depression, PPOCD, and other perinatal mood disorders have intrusive thoughts and are horrified by them, women with PPP are not. They consider their intrusive thoughts rational and are apt to act on them. They experience rapid mood swings, from depression to irritability to euphoria, and lose touch with reality. Women with postpartum psychosis don't believe that anything is wrong with them.

Postpartum psychosis is considered a mental health emergency and requires immediate attention. Women with PPP are at high risk for suicide and infanticide and pose a grave threat to themselves and to their babies. Because women who suffer from the psychosis are not always willing or able to speak with someone about their condition, it's often up to their partner or another family member to help them get the medical attention they need. The condition is usually treated with medications, such as antipsychotic drugs and sometimes antidepressants or antianxiety drugs. If a woman is thought to pose a threat to herself or others, she will likely be hospitalized for a short time. Many women also benefit from psychological counseling and group therapy. With proper care, most women are able to recover from their disorder.

> *"I felt fine. I thought the world had gone mad. Whenever I heard sirens, I thought they were coming to get me. I was sure I only had the flu and since I was the Virgin Mary, God would make me well. When I 'awoke,' so to speak, I was horrified by flashbacks of those thoughts, felt burdened by guilt, and torturously depressed. I felt death would be the only relief. Now I feel like I did come back from the dead."*
>
> —Karen F.

Again, it's important to point out that postpartum psychosis is very rare. To put this condition into context, Andrea Yates, the woman who drowned her five children in the bathtub because she believed if she didn't they would be tormented by Satan, had postpartum psychosis. Research shows that women with a history of **psychosis**, **bipolar disorder**, or **schizophrenia** have a higher risk for developing it.

THE HISTORY OF POSTPARTUM MOOD DISORDERS

POSTPARTUM MOOD disorders, especially postpartum psychosis, have been recognized since ancient times. In 700 BC, Hippocrates described in great detail the emotional problems associated with childbearing that women experienced. The writings of the Greek physician Galen (129–200 AD) and others also mention postpartum emotional problems. But research and study of maternal mental health didn't begin until 1838, when the publication of two volumes by Jean Etienne Dominique Esquirol, linking negative emotional reactions with childbirth, sparked interest in the topic in France. There was a drop in studies during the first half of the twentieth century, but the second half brought an increase in research among the disciplines of psychology, biology, anthropology, and sociology as they related to maternal mental health. In the United States, Dr. James Hamilton (1907–1997) dedicated his career to bringing professional attention to the importance of this topic. In 1962 he wrote *Postpartum Psychiatric Problems*, and thirty years later he coedited *Postpartum Psychiatric Illness: A Picture Puzzle.*

While Dr. Hamilton and many European scientists did much to further our knowledge of postpartum mood disorders, postpartum depression was virtually unheard of, particularly in the United States, until rather recently. For many years, women with PPD and other postpartum mood disorders were considered "manic depressive," or believed to be suffering from "dementia," "toxic confusion," or in a "neurotic state." Most early psychiatrists did not believe that postpartum depression existed as a syndrome separate from major depression, or the clinical depression that many people suffer from at some time in their lives, and that belief has been slow to change in the medical community. In fact, there is still controversy about how to define and classify the depression that occurs in the postpartum period. The second edition of *The Diagnostic and Statistical Manual of Mental Disorders (DSM-II)*, published by the American Psychiatric Association in 1968, described postpartum depression as a separate entity from major depression. But the *DSM-III*, published in 1980, eliminated PPD as a separate category, because it was believed that there was not enough scientific evidence to support the idea that PPD was different from major depression. Postpartum depression is still not recognized by the current *Diagnostic and Statistical Manual of Mental Disorders (DSM-IV)* as being diagnostically distinct from major depression, but it has added a postpartum-onset specifier for patients who develop depression within four weeks of delivery. This means the *DSM-IV* criteria for diagnosing major depression apply to the diagnosis of postpartum depression as well.

In recent years the medical community has begun to focus more intensely on mood disorders related to childbirth, and research on the topic has increased rapidly. We still don't know the exact cause of postpartum depression, but scientists are working to crack the mystery, and their latest research findings continue to improve our ability to recognize and treat PPD and other perinatal mood disorders (see chapter 11 for more information on current research).

Public awareness on the topic has grown rapidly as well. There are several organizations that offer support to women and families going through postpartum mood disorders, making help easier than ever to find. Dr. Hamilton was a cofounder of a scientific organization called the Marcé Society, which he formed in 1980 and named for the early nineteenth-century French doctor, Louis Marcé, who published on the subject in 1858. The Marcé Society has held biennial international conferences on PPD and related disorders since 1984 and works hard to promote public and professional awareness of postpartum mood disorders. Depression After Delivery, the first nonprofit organization of its kind, was founded in 1985 by Nancy Berchtold after she experienced postpartum psychosis. D.A.D.'s mission was to promote universal awareness of mood and anxiety disorders surrounding pregnancy and childbirth and to make known the importance of prevention, early detection, and intervention. In 2005, D.A.D. merged with Postpartum Support International (PSI) to provide information and support to an even wider range of people.

These organized efforts to educate and aid the public, coupled with some of the recent news stories on the topic (in particular, the story of postpartum psychosis sufferer Andrea Yates, who was found not guilty by reason of insanity in July 2006 for drowning her five children in 2001) have helped people see that postpartum depression is a very real and serious problem. In turn, more women are reaching out for help and being diagnosed with PPD than ever before, which means fewer women are suffering needlessly. We believe that this encouraging trend can only continue to get stronger as postpartum depression becomes more mainstream and women begin talking about it and sharing their experiences with others.

Postpartum Depression Is Still Largely Misunderstood

Unfortunately, the medical community has a long history of misunderstanding and misdiagnosing postpartum depression. PPD has traditionally been seen as a condition unrelated to the physical ailments of pregnancy or childbirth, or simply as "regular" depression that just so happens to strike women after they give birth. The medical community is slowly accepting that postpartum depression and major depression are two separate conditions and need to be treated differently, but this old belief is a key reason why PPD has rarely been written about in detail in medical and nursing books and why it's been neglected in medical schools.

Many health-care professionals have been taught to expect a certain degree of emotional upheaval during the postpartum period and are not equipped to recognize postpartum depression and offer help. This has led to a tendency to dismiss new mothers' concerns, brushing them off as hormonal shifts and adjustment to motherhood. This has also led many health-care providers to confuse postpartum depression with the baby blues and tell women that their feelings are normal and will pass when in fact they have PPD. This leads women to be even more hesitant to reach out for help, because they've already been brushed off once.

The traditional belief is that postpartum depression occurs within two or three weeks after giving birth, but recent research has shown that symptoms often don't appear until several months after delivery. Physicians who are unaware of this research often fail to diagnose PPD when it shows up later.

Some health-care practitioners believe that PPD will go away on its own, which is not true. Medication, psychotherapy, or both are needed to make a full recovery. There are still other health-care practitioners who don't take PPD seriously and won't attempt to treat it unless the woman is suicidal, which is a huge mistake. You don't need to be suicidal to be seriously depressed.

The medical community isn't the only place where postpartum depression is misunderstood. Society has traditionally viewed motherhood as a time of pure happiness and joy, which is a completely antiquated notion, but one that has been difficult to change. This unrealistic view of what motherhood should be makes it very difficult for women to admit that they're unhappy and having a hard time. When mothers do express feelings of ambivalence, fear, or rage, they often frighten themselves and those close to them. This has fostered a lack of awareness about postpartum depression among women and the rest of the public.

This lack of awareness and accessible information on PPD has made it difficult for women who have postpartum depression to realize that they can get help to overcome the way they are feeling. Many women strive to meet their own high expectations of motherhood, and when they fall short they are besieged with feelings of inadequacy, guilt, and enormous grief. They believe they feel this way because they are bad mothers, when in reality they are suffering from postpartum depression or some other postpartum mood disorder. They become even more hesitant to reach out for help, and many never end up getting the help that they need.

The good news is that medical research and public discourse about postpartum depression is on the rise. There is more information and help available for women with postpartum depression than ever before, and we are well on our way to rectifying the lingering misunderstandings about this very common condition.

TWO

Understanding PPD Symptoms

ONE OF THE main reasons why postpartum depression can be difficult to diagnose is that there is a wide range of symptoms you can experience, and the severity of those symptoms can differ from woman to woman. Some women look back after being diagnosed and realize that their symptoms began during their pregnancy and became worse after delivery. In fact, 50 percent of postpartum depressions begin during pregnancy. Other women have perfectly normal pregnancies and develop symptoms in the weeks or months after they give birth. Recognizing the onset of PPD can be confusing as well—some of the symptoms, like exhaustion, are normal for new mothers. Others, like mood swings and crying, are associated with the baby blues and could very well pass in a few weeks. In this chapter we describe the symptoms related to postpartum depression and offer tips for coping whenever possible. Keep in mind that these tips are not meant to take the place of your health-care practitioner's advice. They are techniques that we hope will make living with and working through your PPD a little easier and should be used in conjunction with your health-care practitioner's treatment plan. If you haven't seen your health-care practitioner yet and you've experienced any of these symptoms for more than two weeks, or if you feel your symptoms are simply intolerable, make an appointment today.

Mood Swings

Mood swings are extreme changes in mood in brief periods of time. If you feel fine one minute and then suddenly you're hit with a wave of sadness, anxiety, or anger, you're experiencing a mood swing. They are unpredictable and uncontrollable, and their severity can wax and wane. Mood swings are a symptom of hormonal imbalance, so it's not unusual for you to experience them in the first few weeks after giving birth as your hormones adjust. But if you continue to have mood swings for more than two weeks, they could be a warning sign of PPD.

> *"I cried hysterically when I arrived at the zoo and saw that my friend had brought her youngest child. I had only brought my two older kids. It hadn't occurred to me to bring my baby. Why should it? But I cried because it hadn't."*
>
> —Erin T.

There are a few steps you can take to help try to stabilize your mood swings. First, try incorporating exercise into your daily routine. We're not talking about serious cardio—just fifteen minutes of walking each day can elevate your mood and may help ease your mood swings. Make sure you're eating as healthfully as possible, as good nutrition can also work to even out your moods. This may be difficult to do in the first few months with your new baby, but if possible, take a few minutes every two hours to close your eyes and relax. Think of it as your time to reenergize. This will help you relieve stress on a regular basis throughout the day, which in turn can minimize mood swings.

Sadness

Having a baby is a huge life change, so mourning the loss of your old life, your old self, and your freedom is natural. Feelings of sadness are bound to surface in the months after giving birth as you adjust to your new life and learn to see yourself in a new way. It is a part of the normal transition that every mother goes through. For weeks after Sue gave birth, she found herself constantly wishing she could have her old life back. She felt completely unprepared for how drastically her life had changed and wondered if she had made a mistake having a baby.

So while having moments of sadness here and there is normal, if you find yourself feeling sad most of the time, or if your sadness has deepened to despair, you need to call your health-care practitioner. Overwhelming feelings of sadness or persistent sadness that lasts longer than two weeks are big red flags that indicate you probably have postpartum depression.

One way to cope with sadness on your own is to make a list of things that are making you sad. Some of those things will probably be out of your control, but you may be able to do something about the others. For instance, if you're feeling isolated from your friends now that you've had a baby, resolve to make a greater effort and call them twice a week, or plan a get-together once a month. Taking control of even one source of sadness can go a long way toward improving your outlook.

Anxiety

All new mothers are somewhat anxious. How could we not be? Being a new mother means a new job, new responsibilities, a new life—all very good reasons to feel a little worried! We are recovering from childbirth, trying to take care of ourselves, and now suddenly we are completely responsible for another human life. None of us have been trained to be mothers, yet somehow we are expected to know exactly what to do and how to do it. Plus, once you have a newborn of your own, you realize how fragile and vulnerable they are. They can get hurt so easily, and protecting them can seem like an enormous (and even impossible) job. But sometimes women can worry *too* much and their anxiety begins to interfere with their daily activities. Women with severe anxiety are constantly worried that something is wrong with their babies or that they're going to do something wrong or hurt their babies. Many worry about whether they will be able to be good mothers. They can't relax, even when their babies are asleep or someone else is caring for them.

Although much of what happens in the world is out of your control, there are steps you can take to ensure your child's safety and ease your mind at least a little bit. You can make sure that your child is always buckled into his car seat properly; eats enough healthy, nutritious food; visits his pediatrician on a regular basis; gets the proper vaccinations; and so forth. Focusing on what you *can* control in your child's life can help take your mind off the things you can't control.

Panic Attacks

A panic attack is a sudden surge of overwhelming fear that comes without warning and without any obvious reason. It's far more intense than having anxiety or the feeling of being "stressed out" that most people experience. Panic attacks are the most extreme form of anxiety. They can last anywhere from a few minutes to a few hours and may occur once in a while or quite frequently. Here's a list of the physical symptoms associated with panic attacks:

- shaking
- feeling that your heart is pounding or racing
- sweating
- chest pain
- shortness of breath
- feeling that you are choking
- nausea
- cramping
- dizziness

- out-of-body feeling, or feeling surreal
- tingling or numb feeling in your hands
- chills or hot flashes
- knots in your stomach
- feeling like you are "jumping out of your skin"

It's also common to have an extreme fear of losing control, going crazy, or dying during a panic attack. Some women are able to identify what triggers their attacks, such as driving a car or bathing their babies, but for many women panic attacks strike completely out of the blue. Sometimes just the fear of having a panic attack is enough to trigger one. This is the basis for a condition called agoraphobia. If you suffer from agoraphobia, you find it hard to leave home (or another safe area), because you are afraid of having a panic attack in public or not having an easy way to escape if the symptoms start. Panic attacks are truly a terrifying experience and are often mistaken for heart attacks or strokes, which share many of the same symptoms.

> *"I started having panic attacks on the highway. I would suddenly become afraid that I would crash or a truck would hit my car. That's when I decided it was time to get help."*
>
> —Sara L.

There are few strategies you can use to help cope with panic attacks. The first one is called relaxation breathing. Sit or lie down in a comfortable spot and close your eyes. Begin to focus on your breathing and put everything else out of your mind. Now start to pace your breathing by counting with each inhale and exhale—*in-2-3* and *out-2-3*. Gradually take deeper and deeper breaths until you're filling your lungs to capacity with each breath. Continue breathing like this for ten minutes, or until your feeling of panic passes.

Muscle relaxation is often used in conjunction with relaxation breathing. Again, sit or lie down in a comfortable spot and close your eyes. Now mentally scan your body, starting with your toes and working your way slowly up through your legs, buttocks, torso, arms, hands, fingers, neck, and head. Focus on each part individually. Wherever you feel tension, imagine it melting away. Next, tighten the muscles in one area of your body. Hold the muscles for a count of five or more before relaxing and moving on to the next area. This is a good method for releasing tension. Tighten the muscles of your face, shoulders, arms, legs, and buttocks. Make sure to breathe slowly and deeply through the process. Once you feel relaxed, imagine you're in your favorite place or in a spot of great beauty and peacefulness. Stay like this for five to ten minutes before slowly getting up.

You might also want to try a similar strategy called deep breathing. Inhale for four counts, hold your breath for three counts, and then exhale for four counts—*in-2-3-4, hold-2-3,* and *out-2-3-4.* This method enables you to control your breathing so that you can relax. Deep breathing is very handy, because you can practice it anywhere, at any time. In fact, to reap the greatest benefits from deep breathing, you should make it part of your everyday life. Do it while you're driving, grocery shopping, eating dinner, or watching TV. Even one minute of deep breathing can help you feel more in control.

Heavy muscle exercise can also help. Do a couple of push-ups or some standing push-ups, where you place your hands on a wall, elbows bent, and push your body away from the wall. You could also do a full body stretch, reaching your arms as high in the air as you can, or a quick tightening of all the muscles in your body and then releasing them. Try grabbing your steering wheel as tightly as you can while parked or at a stoplight and then releasing your fingers.

Yoga, meditation, and guided imagery are also effective ways to cope with panic attacks. There are lots of good books and tapes available if you're interested in trying them. See the Resources section for some suggestions.

Crying

There are a lot of valid reasons to cry during your postpartum period. The tears can come from feeling overwhelmed, tired, or frustrated. They can stem from the sadness you may be feeling about the loss of your old life, the way you delivered your baby if things didn't go as you planned, or those extra pounds you may still be carrying after your pregnancy. Sometimes having a good cry for no reason just makes you *feel* better. Crying releases stress, and that's a good thing. In fact, crying is actually encouraged by many therapists. But if you find that you're crying more often than not and have no control over your crying, then you may have crossed the line into excessive crying, and that's a problem. Aside from indicating that you're feeling pretty low, excessive crying gets in the way of taking care of yourself and your baby. From her first days your baby is in tune with how you're feeling, and excessive crying can have a negative impact on her development if you don't get treatment (see chapter 8 for more information).

> *"I felt like I couldn't stop crying. Any little thing would set me off. I literally spent hours every day in tears."*
> —Jackie C.

One strategy for coping with crying spells is to allow yourself a specific time during the day to have one. We know this sounds strange, but if crying is one of your milder symptoms and you can control it, this allows you the release that your body and mind need without getting in the way of taking care of your baby or your daily responsibilities. Give yourself fifteen minutes to let it all out while your baby naps, at the end of the day after you've put her to bed, or when your partner is home and can take care of the baby while you're in another room. Another good time to cry is while you're taking a shower. If you have a friend or relative who has had postpartum depression or some other perinatal mood disorder, you could cry to her if you feel comfortable doing so. But you should be confident that she will be very supportive and accepting. The last thing you need is someone making you feel even worse.

Confusion and Difficulty Concentrating

It's common for new mothers to feel a little scatterbrained. You may find that you keep losing your train of thought, or forgetting what you were about to say or do. You may be indecisive, easily distracted, and have trouble making decisions about even the simplest things. You find yourself starting one task, then losing track and beginning another task, like Monique T., who said, "I would go to the linen closet for toilet paper, notice the towels were a mess, straighten them up, and then walk away without the toilet paper. I would walk into a room and get so easily distracted." This state of mind is most likely caused by fatigue, changing hormones, and the stress of your new job as a parent.

Thankfully, there are several things you can do to help sharpen your focus and keep confusion at bay. Make sure that you're getting adequate rest by taking naps when your baby is sleeping, or if that's not possible, taking rest breaks throughout the day. Do your best to eat a healthy diet. Good nutrition will give you energy and help clear your mind. Healthy eating is also vitally important if you are breast-feeding your baby, as you're sharing your nutrients with him at every feeding. Another way to remain focused is to make lists of things you need or want to do. Make your list first thing every morning or every night before you go to bed, and keep it in a place where you spend a lot of time, like your kitchen or your baby's room. That way you can add to it on a continuous basis as you think of tasks and cross off what you've already accomplished. Finally, don't try to do too many things at once. Focus on accomplishing only one task at a time and let the others go.

Irritability and Hypersensitivity

Changing hormones, fatigue, and the stress of being a new mom can also make you irritable and hypersensitive. You're probably feeling very vulnerable right now, and situations and comments that you had no problem letting roll off your back before you had your baby may now cause you a lot of pain or simply just rub you the wrong way.

Your best bet is to explain your feelings to the people around you and ask them to try to be sensitive to your needs. Your partner, family, and friends almost certainly have no idea you're feeling this way, and talking to them about it will help avoid some unpleasant situations as well as strengthen your support network. You should also talk with other moms—most of them will be able to identify with how you're feeling and can reassure you.

Feeling Overwhelmed

Taking care of your new baby (especially if this is your first child) and adjusting to your new life can be quite overwhelming. Many women feel like they no longer have control over their lives, or that they can never get anything done. You have just taken on a *huge* task, and the first thing you need to do is understand that *there is nothing wrong with you for feeling overwhelmed from time to time.* Virtually every new mother has moments when she feels powerless and has trouble coping. But some women spend *most* of their time feeling overwhelmed by their situation and unable to cope, to the point where they become paralyzed by it and can't care for themselves or their babies properly.

One way to combat feeling overwhelmed is to take firm control over what you *can* control. Start with a small task and commit to doing it every day. For instance, you could decide that every day you're going to take a shower or you're going to do one load of dishes. If you can identify exactly what is causing you to feel overwhelmed, start taking baby steps toward fixing it. For example, if you're feeling really overwhelmed by the idea of getting up every two or three hours to breast-feed your baby, pump extra milk during the day and have your partner do the night feedings.

Joyce coaches her patients to take a "pause" from life when they are feeling overwhelmed. Close your eyes and take a few good, deep breaths (see the deep breathing exercise on page 32 for specific instructions) for one minute. If your mind starts racing or thoughts keep popping up, visualize the numbers as you breathe (*in-2-3-4, hold-2-3,* and *out-2-3-4*). Most of her patients are surprised by how much better they feel when they're done.

This is also a good time to take stock of the resources available to you. Could you afford to hire someone to come over and clean your house until you feel in better control of things? Could you order takeout one or two days a week so that you don't have to cook as often? Could your mother or a close friend or relative come over once or twice a week to help you do laundry or clean up the house? This is the time to take advantage of the help that's available to you. Trust us, your friends and family will be happy to do anything they can to make things better for you. Don't be afraid to ask them for help. Joyce wrote herself the following note, which she read at least five times a day when she was going through PPD, to help see this more clearly: "It is hard to say 'help me.' It is even harder not to." Perhaps these words or a similar kind of note will help you to see the importance of asking for help and to feel better about doing it.

Feelings of Inadequacy

Lots of women wrestle with feelings of inadequacy once they get home with their babies. When Sue got home from the hospital, she felt completely inadequate because she couldn't figure out how to get her son to stop crying. For the first three weeks, nothing worked. Then one day she rocked him in a slightly different way, and suddenly he calmed down. It turned out that he wanted Mommy to gently bounce him up and down and not sway from side to side. Despite what you may have heard, being a parent is a *learned* skill. You are not born with an innate ability to mother. It takes time to learn the ropes and figure out how to meet your particular baby's needs.

> *"Everyone says it comes naturally, but it doesn't. Everyone says you're supposed to recognize what your baby's cries mean. I didn't for a long time and I felt so stupid."*
>
> —Neava R.

The best thing you can do to help ease your feelings of inadequacy is to talk with other mothers. When you hear other women talk about their struggles and triumphs, it can give you a sense of hope and shows you that you won't feel inadequate forever. If you don't have any friends with children that you can call, join a new mothers support group or a Mommy and Me group, go to your local library's story hour, or sign up for a postpartum exercise class. There are many organized groups for moms and their babies—do a search on the Internet, call your local YMCA, or ask your pediatrician for some leads. You may have to try several different activities before you find the right fit for you and your baby, but it's definitely worth the effort.

Anger

If you're feeling angry, it's most likely because your expectations about being a mother have not been met. By this point you've probably realized that a lot of things didn't turn out like you thought they would. Perhaps your delivery didn't go the way you wanted it to, your baby doesn't act like you thought he would, you haven't lost your pregnancy weight like you were supposed to, your partner is not helping you the way he or she should—the list is endless. You may also be angry that people are no longer paying attention to you, including your partner. When you were pregnant, *you* were the focus of attention. Everyone was concerned with how you were feeling and how things were going. Now the focus is on the baby, and people may not seem to notice that you are not doing so well. Another common reason women feel angry is that although their life has changed dramatically, it seems like their partner's life is the same as it always was.

> *"I felt like my life changed so drastically and my husband's was the same. At least he could leave, be with grown-ups, take a break, get paid, feel productive, have fun, sit down during meals, go to the bathroom alone, get dressed, knows his job comfortably well, and was not alone like I was. I was really pissed."*
>
> —Jessie L.

It's important that you don't try to ignore your anger. Instead, you need to try to find constructive ways of expressing it. For instance, you could begin keeping a journal and write out all your angry thoughts and feelings. Or you could try expressing it physically by screaming in the shower or punching a pillow. Just be careful not to let your anger become destructive. Samantha K. got so angry one day that she punched a hole in her kitchen wall. Not only did she hurt herself, but she also scared both her partner and her baby and wound up feeling horribly guilty about her outburst. Exercise is also a great way to release your anger and elevate your mood. Take every opportunity you can to go for a walk or hit the gym. Make your anger work for you. Kellie G. progressed from kicking a cardboard box in her basement to an exercise routine that changed her whole lifestyle.

If you need a way to dissolve your anger quickly, try removing yourself from the situation, even for a moment. Leave the room, go outside and walk around your house, get a glass of water, do a push-up, or wash your hands.

You also need to figure out constructive ways to talk about your anger. It's so easy to lash out at the people you love when you're angry, but as you may have already discovered, you just wind up feeling worse if you do. Try counting to ten before you address what has made you angry. That may be all you need to help you speak calmly and avoid putting the other person on the defensive. Be direct, and try not to be accusatory when you're talking. Instead of saying, "You made me so mad when you came home late last night. You are so inconsiderate!" tell your partner, "I felt upset and angry when you worked late last night. I really needed a break from the baby."

Keep in mind that your partner may be angry as well. Surely he had expectations about being a parent that haven't been met as well, so you should be prepared to hear about his anger and acknowledge it. Sometimes it's enough just to get the anger off your chest, even if there's nothing you or anyone else can do about it.

Guilt

Until you've had a baby, it's difficult to understand how big a role guilt can play in a mother's life. Working moms feel guilty for not spending enough time with their children. Stay-at-home moms feel guilty for wanting to take a break from their babies each day, or conversely, for spending *too* much time with them. Maybe you feel guilty because you can't seem to balance your old life and obligations with your new one. Or perhaps you feel guilty when you're doing the housework and your baby is left in his bouncer to occupy himself. Or maybe one or more of these situations is the source of your guilt:

- You're still carrying extra baby weight
- You had a C-section instead of a vaginal delivery
- You did not conceive "naturally"
- You feel completely inexperienced and overwhelmed
- You had a girl but your partner wanted a boy
- You can't handle everything alone
- You feel resentment toward your baby for changing your life
- You're not breast-feeding
- You don't want to have sex
- You have to take medication for your PPD
- You don't think you're bonding with your baby properly
- You don't love every minute of motherhood
- You resent getting up every two hours at night
- You don't understand your baby's cries yet
- You're bored with the repetition of staying home with your baby and would rather work

The list goes on and on. The point here is that all mothers feel guilt about *something,* big or small.

When you have postpartum depression, sometimes your symptoms themselves can cause you to feel guilty. For instance, women who have intrusive thoughts (see page 44 for more information) usually feel extremely guilty about having them. And the very fact that you are not the glowing, happy, well-adjusted new mother that society "expects" you to be can cause a lot of guilt. Know this: You do not have postpartum depression because you did something wrong. You have a medical illness, and you do not have to feel guilty for feeling like you do.

One way to get past some of your guilt is to try reasoning with yourself. If you have to work to help support your family, you're not choosing to work over staying at home with your baby—it's a necessity. Millions of babies are in day care or have someone other than their parents taking care of them on a daily basis, and those babies turn out just fine.

Monitoring your self-talk is also important when trying to cope with your guilty feelings. If you're constantly telling yourself that you're not a good mother because you work all day and your baby is in day care, or that you're a bad person for neglecting your partner in order to take care of your baby, it's only going to compound your guilt. Concentrate on the positive as much as you can. For instance, congratulate yourself for finding the best possible day-care center for your baby, and think about the good things about day care, such as how your child will get to socialize and make friends much earlier than if you were staying at home with her.

Finally, talk to other moms. As we emphasized above, all moms feel guilt about something and can completely relate to how you're feeling. Often another mom can reassure you better than anyone that your feelings of guilt are common.

Sleep Problems

Sleep deprivation is a huge problem and one that should be addressed immediately. Mothers with newborns need at least four hours of good, uninterrupted sleep in order to function and feel reasonably well. There are several different kinds of sleep problems that women can experience, and all of them result in sleep deprivation.

Insomnia is pretty self-evident—you're having difficulty getting any sleep at all. If you find yourself lying awake at night fretting about your baby, what you have to do, what you think you *should* be doing, and so on, then anxiety and worry are most likely the sources of your insomnia. In addition to the tips we offer below, see page 29 for advice on coping with anxiety.

Difficulty falling asleep is also linked to anxiety. The relaxation techniques we describe in the panic attacks section on page 30 may help you take your mind off your worries and fall asleep more quickly.

Oversleeping, or sleeping *too* much, is a classic sign of depression. Women who oversleep have a very hard time getting up when they need to, such as for night feedings or in the morning when their babies are ready to start the day, and they find themselves napping at every possible opportunity.

Women who have early morning wakings are waking up *too* early—before they've gotten enough sleep and before their babies need to be fed or are rising for the day themselves.

Having difficulty falling back asleep after being awoken is also quite common with new mothers, especially after waking up to feed your baby in the night.

Here are some healthy sleep guidelines that may ease the sleep problems described above.

1. Night feedings aside, try to go to bed and wake up at roughly the same time every day. This can help get your body back on schedule.
2. Don't consume caffeinated products like coffee, tea, soda, or chocolate.
3. Certain medications can interfere with your ability to sleep. Check with your health-care practitioner to see if any of the prescription drugs you're taking may be the culprit.
4. Exercise as early in the day as possible.
5. Make your bedroom your sleep sanctuary. In other words, don't watch TV, read, or play with your baby there. Your bedroom should be only for sleep.
6. Don't eat anything in the two to three hours before bedtime.
7. Make an effort to relax before bedtime. Dim the lights, put your feet up, and unwind a little before getting into bed. Or soak in the bath with a magazine.
8. If you can't fall asleep within twenty to thirty minutes, don't lie there tossing and turning. Get out of bed and go into another room to read or listen to quiet music for a while.
9. Don't look at your clock. Watching it will only increase your anxiety and insomnia.
10. Nap during the day when your baby naps or when someone is there to watch him for you. If you can't nap, then at least rest.

Fatigue

Low energy and fatigue are usually caused by hormonal imbalances and the sleep deprivation that new mothers experience when they get home with their babies. How long you'll feel fatigued is often influenced by the physical shape you're in and what type of birth experience you had. Women who've had a Caesarean section or have fussier-than-normal or colicky babies often feel fatigued longer than those who had normal vaginal deliveries or have calmer, quieter babies. Fatigue can also be exacerbated by insomnia, breast-feeding, a weak support system, the recycling of hormones during the postpartum period, a busy schedule, and too many visitors.

The first thing you should do is ask your health-care practitioner to give you a physical and do blood work to rule out any underlying illnesses, such as hypothyroidism (see page 54 in chapter 3 for more information on hypothyroidism).

If hypothyroidism is not the culprit, there are a few things you can do to increase your energy and fight off fatigue. Use the time your baby is napping to get some sleep yourself, or if you can't sleep, put your feet up and take a rest. You could read a magazine, watch TV, knit—anything that you find relaxing and *not* a chore.

Exercise is also a very effective way to increase your energy. We know it can be difficult to motivate yourself to exercise when you're bone tired, but it really works. Try taking your baby out for a walk every morning, or arrange for your partner or a family member or friend to watch your baby so you can hit the gym a few times a week. Many fitness centers also have on-site babysitting services, if you feel comfortable using one. YMCAs usually have mother and baby swimming or gym classes that you could try. Whatever you choose to do, try to get in at least one half hour of activity five times a week.

Eating a good diet can make a big difference when it comes to your energy level. Focus on eating more whole grains, lean protein, vegetables, and fruit. Keep healthy snacks like granola bars, yogurt, and baby carrots on hand to help you avoid reaching for sugary treats. Make sure you remain hydrated by drinking water throughout the day.

Changes in Appetite

Many women either find themselves battling sudden cravings or losing their appetite all together. Sue remembers having no appetite at all for weeks after her son was born. The thought of food was distasteful to her, and she essentially munched on Honey Nut Cheerios all day. She lost all of her baby weight in three weeks, but her milk production suffered badly, and her son wound up losing weight instead of gaining it. This, of course, exacerbated all of the other PPD symptoms she was experiencing, like crying, anxiety, and feeling overwhelmed.

You need to fuel your body to stay healthy, feel good, and provide your baby with the proper nutrients while breast-feeding. Do your best to eat six mini-meals per day or three regular meals with two wholesome snacks in between. High-protein foods, such as yogurt, cheese, and oatmeal, are good choices. Joyce snacked on banana slices smeared with peanut butter to keep her strength up. Also be sure to drink plenty of water or Gatorade, which will help replace your body's electrolytes.

The best way to deal with cravings is to allow yourself to indulge, but do it *in moderation*. If you're craving cookies, take one or two out of the box and put the box back in your cupboard, out of sight, so you're not tempted to eat more. You need to satisfy your cravings or they'll get worse, but you should be very mindful of empty calories you're consuming.

If you're struggling because you have no appetite, it's very important to try to find some foods that appeal to you. Good nutrition is crucial to both your physical and emotional health, and if you're breast-feeding it becomes even more important. As Sue's story above demonstrates, when you don't eat enough, you run the risk of being unable to produce enough milk to feed your baby properly. That knowledge alone should be enough to get you back to the refrigerator. Ann Dunnewold and Diane Sanford offer a great idea in their book *Postpartum Survival Guide*. They suggest you think about the comfort foods you loved as a kid—macaroni and cheese, grilled cheese sandwiches, chicken soup—and see if they spark your appetite. If you simply can't bring yourself to eat, you should seek professional help immediately.

Intrusive Thoughts

Intrusive thoughts are bizarre, uncharacteristic thoughts that pop into your head out of nowhere. Oftentimes these thoughts center on your baby's fragility. Newborns certainly *look* fragile and need to be handled with care, but it usually doesn't take long for new mothers to realize that they're sturdier than they look and to get accustomed to holding, bathing, and changing them. However, many women who suffer from postpartum depression begin to have intrusive thoughts about doing something to hurt their babies. For instance, you could be giving your baby a bath and suddenly think, "I could just let her head slip under water and drown her." Intrusive thoughts can cause a lot of anxiety, because it's scary to realize that you're capable of thinking (but never doing) these types of things. It's very important to note that women with PPD *never* act on intrusive thoughts.

> *"I was cutting up chicken to cook for dinner when I suddenly imagined cutting up my baby. I was terrified."*
> —Yolanda M.

Intrusive thoughts are a symptom of postpartum depression—they are caused by your illness, not by a desire to hurt your baby. Women with PPD are frightened by their intrusive thoughts, but they understand that such thoughts are completely out of the realm of reality and would never carry them out. Women with postpartum psychosis, however, are usually not afraid of these thoughts and consider them viable and rational. This makes them a very grave risk to themselves and their children.

A good way to put this in perspective is to understand that intrusive thoughts are common and normal for everyone—men and women—at any time in our lives. Here's a good example: A few years ago, Joyce was driving down the road and saw a man on a bicycle riding up ahead of her. Suddenly she thought, *What if I hit him? Will he go over the guardrail and into the river?* Joyce knew she would never do it and felt no guilt about her thought. In fact, she was excited that she had a good non-PPD-related intrusive thought to share with her patients. The difference between the intrusive thoughts we have in regular life and the ones spurred on by PPD is that we feel no guilt or anxiety about the ones we have in regular life. We feel secure in the knowledge that we would never act on these strange thoughts. We see them for what they are—anomalies that have no bearing on the kind of people we are. When you have PPD, you still know that you would never do anything to harm your child, but the illness makes you feel fearful and anxious about the thoughts themselves. The illness makes you doubt yourself and feel afraid that there is something wrong with you for thinking these types of things.

If you're having intrusive thoughts, it's very important for you to share them with someone who is nonjudgmental and extremely understanding, such as a therapist, who can normalize them for you. Intrusive thoughts are the most difficult PPD symptom to treat and get past, because they hurt the very core of your soul as a person and mother. It can be difficult to forgive yourself for these thoughts, but you must in order to recover from postpartum depression and move on. A therapist is the best person to help you do this.

Shame

Feeling shame because you're suffering from postpartum depression is often the biggest roadblock to getting better, because it prevents you from reaching out for help when you need it. It's easy to see why we might be ashamed to admit we have PPD. It's been a long-held belief in our society that all new mothers should be happy, joyful, and relaxed after they have their babies. That's just not true. The reality is that caring for an infant is probably the hardest, most stressful job on earth. This societal myth is truly damaging, because it makes women who are feeling sad, anxious, or overwhelmed to think there's something wrong with them and that they are alone in having these feelings. But know this: *There is no shame in having postpartum depression.*

It is a medical illness. Close to seven hundred thousand women suffer from it each year. It is the most common complication after childbirth. The shame is that women feel they can't admit it when things aren't all rosy for them after they get home with their babies. Shame is the reason why thousands and thousands of women with PPD go untreated for far too long and suffer needlessly. Postpartum depression is the easiest perinatal mood disorder to overcome. All you need to do is take the first step and see your health-care practitioner. Share how you feel with someone you are comfortable with, who will be non-judgmental. After all, you did not cause this to happen. Postpartum depression is a medical illness just as diabetes is, and it requires medical treatment in order for you to recover.

Memory Loss

It's a well-documented fact that depression impairs our ability to form long-term memories, and it's also very common for women to complain of memory loss after delivery. The reason for this memory loss has been traced to a loss of our ability to concentrate and remember because of the illness. Say, for instance, you agreed to meet your friend at a restaurant for lunch. She told you what time to be there, but an hour later you can't remember the agreed-upon time. You haven't really "forgotten" the time—it's just that a lack of concentration prevented you from forming an enduring memory of the time in the first place. It "went in one ear and out the other," so to speak.

A good way to cope with memory loss is to write down important information like dates, times, and addresses as they are told to you. Use one of those large desk calendars to keep track of your schedule, or a daily planner if you want something you can easily carry around with you.

Excessive Concern for Your Baby

Every mother feels concern for her baby's safety, and sometimes we are a little overprotective, especially with a first child. Some women, however, develop a persistent and all-consuming overconcern for their babies' well-being, so much so that it interferes with their daily activities. This behavior is sometimes called overbonding or hypervigilance (unwarranted overconcern). Women who are overly concerned for their babies may be unwilling to leave the house for fear that some harm might come to their baby in the car or in a public place. Some women are overly fearful of "germs," in part because of society's focus on newborns and their perceived susceptibility to illness. Others may feel extreme stress when their babies don't act like they're "supposed" to. For instance, one woman Sue knows became very upset when her baby didn't finish his bottle, because she was worried he wasn't getting enough to eat. Her pediatrician had told her that her baby should be drinking a certain number of ounces of milk each day, so if he didn't hit that mark, even by an ounce or two, she became distraught.

If your overconcern pertains to germs, talk with your pediatrician or other mothers about your feelings. They can help put your concerns in perspective and normalize them for you. The best way to cope with excessive concern for your baby is to discuss them with a therapist so that she can help you work through them.

Disinterest in Your Baby

Many people think that the moment you hold your baby in your arms, you fall in love and form an instant bond with her. But the truth is that it takes time for that special bond to develop. You and your baby need to get to know each other a bit in order for those strong feeling of attachment to take root. It can take more than a few weeks for some women to really begin to feel love for their babies, and that's perfectly normal. But if you find that a month or so has gone by and you have absolutely no interest in your child (also known as underbonding), it's time to consult your health-care practitioner. A long-term lack of interest in your baby is a serious problem for many reasons. Most important, it may affect your ability to take care of her properly, and it can have serious repercussions for her emotional development. Turn to chapter 8 for more information on how postpartum depression can affect your baby.

"I loved my son, but I didn't really like him. I felt detached. He seemed like just a lump of flesh to me."

—Gina T.

The fact is that it's completely normal not to feel instantly bonded to your baby, even though society expects new mothers to do so naturally. The best way to cope with this is to understand that bonding takes time, and the older your baby gets, the closer you will feel to him.

Fear of Harming Yourself

Some moms feel so overwhelmed and depressed over their situation that they occasionally have suicidal ideations, or thoughts of suicide. For women with postpartum depression, that's exactly what they are—just thoughts. They are fleeting feelings that occur when we are in the middle of a crisis and feel helpless and backed into a corner. Postpartum depression is a crisis, and occasional suicidal thoughts, such as *I wish I were dead; it would be easier than this,* are common. Women with PPD usually have no intention of carrying out suicide, so occasional thoughts like this are not cause for alarm. That said, women who express an intention to commit suicide or have a plan to do so require immediate medical intervention. Any thoughts of self-harm should be discussed with a therapist.

"I never thought about harming the baby. I felt before I would do that I would hurt myself."

—Jenn S.

Loss of Interest in Activities, Friends, and Family

Similar to the type of depression that can occasionally occur at other times in our lives, postpartum depression can cause you to lose interest in the hobbies and activities that used to bring you pleasure. For example, Joyce loved music her whole life, but when she developed postpartum depression she stopped listening to it. She suddenly found music irritating and aggravating. You may find that you no longer have any motivation or desire to go to the movies, eat at your favorite restaurant, or go shopping like you used to. Or perhaps you belonged to a club or volunteered somewhere but can't bring yourself to get involved again.

> *"I was obsessed with scrapbooking to the tiniest detail. I enjoyed it and it was therapy for me. I felt proud of what I could accomplish. After I had Alex, I hated it and had no desire to work that hard again. That just wasn't me."*
> —Adele S.

Another classic symptom of depression is decreased socialization, or isolating yourself from your friends and family. You may not want to go to your cousin's wedding on Saturday but feel like you have to, or you may dread your best friend coming over for a visit. Having postpartum depression is scary, and admitting that you feel sad, angry, or overwhelmed can be difficult when you believe you're supposed to be happy. Sometimes it seems easier not to talk to your family and friends when you're living with this huge, all-encompassing unhappiness that you don't want to (or are afraid to) talk about. After all, what is there to say when you can't talk about the elephant in the room? It's also difficult to be interested in anyone else's life when you're going through postpartum depression. You're so absorbed in what's going on with yourself that everything else becomes unimportant. It's hard enough most days to take care of yourself and your baby.

A good way to cope with losing interest in friends, family, and activities is to normalize it. You've just had a baby—no one expects you to jump back into your social life and old activities. It takes time to rebalance your life. You're going through a major period of adjustment and working very hard to master your new role. However, if your disinterest lasts more than a month or two and others begin to voice concern about it, you should talk with a therapist.

Lack of Interest in Sex

The idea of sex is usually the last thing on a new mother's mind in the weeks after childbirth. First of all, your body has just undergone a big trauma, and physically you need to heal before attempting to have sex again. Most obstetricians recommend waiting six to eight weeks after childbirth before resuming your sex life, especially if you've had a Caesarean section. The impact of changing hormones greatly affects the libido. The exhaustion and stress of taking care of a newborn can make it difficult to feel amorous. Many women are fearful of getting pregnant again, and that makes them want to avoid sex. Others feel like the baby is on them all day long, and just don't want to be touched anymore. Mentally, most women do not feel good about the appearance of their bodies after having a baby. On top of all this, taking care of a baby is a twenty-four-hour job, and often it seems impossible just to find enough *time* for sex. But eventually most new moms adjust to their new schedules, their bodies heal, and sex is no longer considered a "chore."

> *"Vicki didn't want to have sex with me, even after six weeks. I didn't think she loved me anymore, or thought I was attractive. I was wrong—I just needed to give her time and understanding. We had to work at it, but eventually Vicki and I reconnected."*
>
> —Ray C.

Although spontaneity is great, it might not be practical with a new baby around, so one way to try sparking your libido is to schedule some time for intimacy. Maybe you don't *consciously* want sex, but if you can make the time and create the mood, you may find that your desire is just hidden under the stress and exhaustion of being a new mom. Drop the baby off at your parents' house if you can, or have a family member or a friend come over and take the baby for a walk. Once you're alone with your partner, do something relaxing, such as take a bath, give each other a massage, or just lie together on your bed. Sometimes all you need is a little peace and closeness to feel ready to try sex again. And even if you find you still have no interest in sex, just being affectionate and spending quality time together may help.

Another idea that has worked for many women is to have a trusted support person watch the baby overnight and go to a hotel for a romantic escape. Getting away from your house and your daily responsibilities can help rekindle your libido.

You and your partner can also try talking together with a therapist to work out your issues.

Somatic Symptoms

There are also several less serious yet still unpleasant physical symptoms of PPD that you may experience, many of which are related to the symptoms already described in this chapter.

Many women with postpartum depression become either constipated or have recurrent diarrhea. There are different causes for these bowel function issues—having a Caesarean section, hemorrhoids from pregnancy, and stress are the most common. If you are constipated, you could try using Feosal, an over-the-counter stool softener, to help alleviate the problem. Many obstetricians instruct their patients to take it to help regulate their bowel movements again after a Caesarean section. If you're having frequent diarrhea, be sure to not only drink a lot of water to keep yourself hydrated, but also to increase the amount of fiber in your diet. In fact, a healthy diet is crucial to maintaining proper bowel function, and regular exercise is also important.

Itchiness is another irritating symptom you may experience. Dry skin is often caused by hormonal changes, but it can also be a response to stress and emotional issues. Buy a deep moisturizer at your local drugstore and rub it on your trouble spots each night before bed. Or better yet, have your partner do it for you.

Sore muscles often plague women with postpartum depression, as stress, anxiety, and other PPD symptoms can increase the tension in your body and creep into your muscles. Stretching, hot baths, and massages all work well to relieve muscle tension.

Other common symptoms include headaches, a sense of restlessness, chest pains, heart palpitations, and hyperventilation. All of these symptoms indicate you are operating under a high level of stress or anxiety, and can mark the beginning of more serious symptoms like panic attacks (see page 30).

THREE

Risk
Factors

No **ONE KNOWS** why some women develop postpartum depression and others do not. What we do know is that a combination of biological, psychological, and social factors work together to increase your risk for developing the condition. In this chapter we describe the factors that can contribute to postpartum depression and offer words of advice for reducing your risk whenever we can.

Why Is Knowing Your Risk Factors Important?

There are several very good reasons for you to determine exactly what your risk factors are for postpartum depression. First, if you're reading this book in an effort to educate yourself on what postpartum period can bring, knowing your risk factors will help you recognize PPD a lot faster if it occurs. Once you know what types of things contribute to the development of PPD, you'll naturally be more aware of how your risk factors are affecting your life after your baby is born. It can also help you preemptively—if you discover that you are at high risk for developing PPD, you can seek out the appropriate help before it occurs.

If you suspect that you have postpartum depression, you need to become an "educated consumer" in order to get the right kind of help for your condition. Knowing your risk factors will enable you to go to your health-care practitioner armed with the information she needs to properly diagnose and treat you.

Finally, since research shows that the combinations of factors that contribute to postpartum depression are different for every woman, you must understand your own personal risk factors in order to work through them. Some risk factors, like heredity or previous depressive episodes, are permanent and unchangeable. But others, such as marital problems or a weak support system, can be improved, and making these improvements will help you feel better more quickly.

Biological Risk Factors

History of Thyroid Problems

The thyroid gland is located on the front part of the neck below the thyroid cartilage (Adam's apple). The gland produces thyroid hormones, which regulate body metabolism. Thyroid hormones are important in regulating body energy, the body's use of other hormones and vitamins, and the growth and maturation of body tissues.

If you have a personal or a family history of thyroid problems, you are at an increased risk for developing postpartum depression. Thyroid problems come in two main forms: hypothyroidism (see page 54 for more information), which is when too little of the thyroid hormone is produced, and hyperthyroidism, which is when too much hormone is produced. It is a very good idea to have baseline blood work done by your physician so you have something with which you can compare any postpartum blood work. This baseline workup should include all thyroid function studies.

Hypothyroidism

After giving birth, sometimes the level of hormones your thyroid produces drops even lower than it was before you got pregnant. This underproduction of thyroid hormones, also known as hypothyroidism, can cause a number of different symptoms, including mood swings, sleep problems, weight gain, irritability, fatigue, and stress. These symptoms can have a significant affect on your emotional well-being and make you more vulnerable to developing postpartum depression.

> *"I felt so tired and lethargic. The doctor told me it was because I was a new mom, and that I should give it time. I gave it time, but I felt worse and worse, so I pushed to have blood work done after speaking to a specialist in PPD. It turned out I had hypothyroidism, and now I'm on Synthroid. I still get exhausted (what new mom doesn't?), but it's not anything like that disabling fatigue I used to feel."*
>
> —Toni A.

It's also important to note that a low thyroid production problem can be exacerbated by your body's increased production of the hormone prolactin. Prolactin is the hormone your body produces to stimulate your milk supply and enable you to breast-feed your baby. Prolactin levels remain high for as long as you nurse your baby, and even women who don't nurse have high prolactin levels for several months after childbirth. It's rare, but occasionally this increase in prolactin production can cause a temporary or permanent condition of low thyroid after pregnancy.

If you're experiencing any of the symptoms listed above, ask your physician to test your thyroid levels. A simple blood test will reveal if there is a problem, and your physician can prescribe medication you can take to restore your thyroid production to the proper levels. Thyroid problems and postpartum depression share many of the same symptoms, and thyroid problems must be ruled out first before you can be diagnosed with postpartum depression.

Breast-feeding and Weaning

There are serious hormonal changes linked to breast-feeding and weaning your baby, and they can put you at a greater risk for developing postpartum depression. The hormone prolactin is produced in great quantity to support nursing, and your prolactin levels remain high until you wean your baby. This accelerated production of prolactin interferes with your body's ability to produce estrogen and progesterone, so your body has trouble replenishing the stores of these two hormones, which pregnancy has depleted. Even when you stop nursing (or if you chose not to nurse), your prolactin levels will remain elevated for months, and normal production of estrogen and progesterone may not resume for a while. In addition, weaning may lead to a drop in your endorphin hormone levels as your prolactin levels return to normal. Have you ever gotten that sudden feeling of peace and contentedness while you were nursing? That's your endorphins kicking in. Without those endorphins circulating through your body, you may find that you feel unhappy when you wean your baby, especially if you do it suddenly. It's best to wean your baby gradually, over a period of a few weeks, if you can.

There are other, non-hormone-related reasons why breast-feeding and weaning can put you at risk. Breast-feeding can be very physically demanding, and some women feel like they spend all of their time nursing. For instance, if your baby needs to eat every two hours and it takes you forty-five minutes to nurse her, then you really don't have the time or even the energy to accomplish anything else. Plus you have virtually no freedom from your baby or time for yourself, which can be hard on you emotionally. Sue had a very difficult time breast-feeding, and it was a big factor in the development of her postpartum depression. Her son was born weighing eleven pounds, and he never seemed to be satisfied after a feeding. He nursed constantly, and sometimes Sue would spend an entire day just sitting on the sofa nursing him. It was utterly exhausting, but her delivery had gone badly and she was determined to get this right. At his three-week pediatrician checkup, Sue learned that her son had lost almost a pound and had to take him to the hospital for tests to make sure he wasn't dehydrated or malnourished. She felt so inadequate—her baby was starving and she had let it happen. After that day, Sue nursed him at every feeding and then gave him a bottle of formula to make sure he wasn't still hungry. She also pumped twice a day to keep her milk supply up. Talk about a lot of work! But she was determined that her baby was going to get as much breast milk as she could give him. In retrospect Sue sees how obsessive this was, and knows that she did it because to *not* do it would have made her feel like a complete failure. She breast-fed for four months, and after she weaned, the situation actually got better for her.

Weaning your baby can be just as difficult as trying to keep up with the emotional demands of feeding her. Many women view breast-feeding as a special time of closeness and bonding with their baby and are sad to give that up. Other women want desperately to breast-feed but can't because they must take certain medications or aren't producing enough milk to nourish their baby. Such situations can make weaning especially difficult, because many of these women already feel like failures, which only aggravates any feelings of inadequacy they may already have as a mom.

Basically, the more important breast-feeding is to you, the more difficult it will be on you emotionally to wean. Whatever your reasons for weaning, the key is to think positively about this new phase in the lives of you and your baby. Negative self-talk about this transition will only make you feel sad and upset, and can open the door even further for PPD.

Complications During Pregnancy or Childbirth

It's difficult to pinpoint the degree to which complications during pregnancy or childbirth contribute to the development of postpartum depression. However, most women agree that difficult pregnancies and birth experiences have a profound effect on them during the postpartum period. Perhaps you had to go on bed rest for the last few months of your pregnancy, or you went into premature labor. Some pregnant women are diagnosed with a non-pregnancy-related illness, such as heart disease. Some women gain a huge amount of weight during pregnancy, and still others experience extreme physical discomfort during their pregnancies. Situations like these can take a big emotional toll at an already vulnerable time in your life. Interestingly, statistics also show that women who visit their physicians more than the standard number of times during pregnancy are more apt to develop PPD.

In the delivery room, it's not uncommon for women who assumed they would have a vaginal birth to suddenly find themselves needing a C-section. That is what happened to Sue when she gave birth to her son. She had chosen to use a midwife and was determined to have as "natural" a birth as possible. She was nine days overdue when her water broke (with a little help from a castor oil/cranberry juice cocktail: not recommended), and her labor pains started a few hours later. She labored all night and finally went to the hospital at 6 AM the next morning. There, Sue sat in a hot shower and did all the things she was taught to do to cope with the pain and help move the birthing process along. Her contractions were somewhat abnormal—there was no break from the pain. It went back and forth from bad to really bad. Six hours later she was only two centimeters dilated. Her midwife suggested she have an epidural in the hope that it would relax her and she would begin to dilate, and Sue agreed. Her biggest fear was having a C-section, and she was prepared to do anything to avoid one. The epidural worked—five hours later Sue was fully dilated and ready to push. Unfortunately, her midwife had underestimated the size of her baby; after an hour and a half of pushing, his heart rate began to drop and it was determined that he was too big to be pushed out. Sue had to be sent into surgery for a C-section. Her eleven-pound baby was born healthy, but that C-section marked the beginning of Sue's postpartum depression. Her birth had gone "wrong," and the symptoms of PPD seemed to follow.

For various reasons, some women unexpectedly have to go through childbirth without their partners there to support them. Other women, most commonly single mothers, don't have someone they feel comfortable asking to support them through their delivery (see page 70 for a detailed discussion on single moms) and think they must go through the experience alone. Sometimes the obstetrician you've come to trust doesn't make it to the delivery, and you have to go through the experience with a stranger. Some babies need special medical attention or surgery after the birth, which can be a nerve-wracking experience. Some women don't discover they're having twins or multiples until they give birth. As you can see, there are a lot of things, big and small, that can happen during your pregnancy and birth experience that can affect your mood postpartum, and much of it has to do with your expectations. Most women, consciously or unconsciously, have set ideas about how they believe their pregnancy and birth experience should be. When the birthing process doesn't go as expected, it can be difficult to adapt, which can lead to feelings of depression and anxiety.

Prior History of Mental Illness

If you've been depressed or had anxiety before, or if you suffer from obsessive-compulsive disorder, you are at an increased risk for postpartum depression. Studies show that women with no history of depression have a 10 percent chance of developing PPD, while women who do have a history have a 25 percent chance. Studies have also shown that a history of depression in your family can increase your chances of developing PPD, and you're at even greater risk if your mother or another relative experienced postpartum depression. Women with bipolar disorder run a very high risk for developing postpartum depression as well—one in five women with bipolar disorder will experience PPD. Bipolar disorder is also a significant risk factor for postpartum psychosis, the rarest and most dangerous type of perinatal mood disorder.

If you haven't done so already, it's a good idea to find out if there's a history of anxiety, depression, or bipolar disorder in your family. Talk to someone you feel comfortable with, anyone who you think may be able to answer your questions. The women in your family, especially your mom, are usually the best place to start. In addition to discussing anxiety, depression, and bipolar disorder in your family tree, ask if your mother or any of your other female relatives had PPD or any kind of postpartum difficulties. You should also ask whether any of the women experienced hormone-related problems like PMS or **premenstrual**

dysphoric disorder or had problems during menopause, as hormones play a role in the development of postpartum depression as well.

Depression or Anxiety During Pregnancy

If you've struggled with depression or anxiety in the past (or to a lesser extent, if they run in your family), you're more likely to become depressed or anxious during your pregnancy. Even if you've never experienced a full-blown bout of depression or acute anxiety but have a tendency to get down or anxious during stressful or uncertain times, you may be more susceptible to depression when you're expecting. In turn, being depressed during your pregnancy is a very strong indicator that you will experience postpartum depression. The symptoms are the same for antepartum and postpartum depression, so you may experience a continuation of the symptoms you had during pregnancy, or they could worsen after the baby is born.

Studies also show that women with previous pregnancy-related depressive episodes are at a 50 to 62 percent increased risk of recurrent episodes with subsequent pregnancies. So if you're pregnant now and were depressed in your previous pregnancy, you should prepare yourself for the possibility that it will happen again. Have a plan of action in place with your health-care practitioner that you can initiate as soon as you begin to feel the symptoms of depression. If you treat your depression during your pregnancy, you have a much better chance of minimizing or even avoiding postpartum depression once your baby is born. If it isn't treated, there's a 50 percent chance your depression will continue or worsen after delivery.

Premenstrual Dysphoric Disorder (PMDD)

Lots of women experience premenstrual syndrome (PMS), or bloating, breast tenderness, and moodiness in the days leading up to their menstrual period. Premenstrual dysphoric disorder (PMDD) is a much more severe premenstrual condition that affects up to 5 percent of women of reproductive age. Like PMS, PMDD often includes physical symptoms, but it always involves a worsening of mood that interferes with a woman's quality of life. Women with PMDD experience symptoms that are very similar to those of postpartum depression in the week before their period, including a depressed mood, anxiety, anger, fatigue, sleep problems, and feelings of being overwhelmed or out of control. PMDD is considered a mood disorder by most medical professionals and is generally treated with antidepressant medication.

Research has shown that women with a personal or family history of depression are at a greater risk of developing PMDD. Likewise, women who suffer from PMDD are at greater risk for developing postpartum depression.

Side Effects from Oral Contraceptives

All oral contraceptives contain hormones, no matter what the dosage, and this means some of them can cause side effects in some women. If you experienced side effects from an oral contraceptive that you've taken in the past, particularly mood-related effects, this puts you at a greater risk for developing postpartum depression. Side effects include mood swings, irritability, sleep problems, decreased concentration, and anger, as well as headaches, migraines, and irregular bleeding.

Previous Postpartum Depression

The single greatest predictor of postpartum depression is a previous episode of postpartum depression. You have approximately a 50 percent chance of developing PPD again with subsequent deliveries if you sought help the first time, and the odds increase even further if you didn't. Katharina Dalton, MD, who did postpartum research in England for about thirty years before she passed away in September 2004, found a 66 percent recurrence rate for women who did not seek treatment for PPD the first time they went through it. The recurrence is generally of the same type, meaning if you had a severe case of postpartum depression the first time, you will have a severe case the next time as well.

The best way to reduce your risk for developing postpartum depression again is to make sure you've made a full physical and emotional recovery from your first episode. You should also figure out a plan of action before your next baby is born to address PPD if it returns. Make sure your health-care practitioner is aware of your previous postpartum depression so he knows to be especially vigilant. Now that you know what your symptoms are and how to recognize the onset of PPD, don't hesitate to call your health-care practitioner if they resurface. If you get treatment quickly, you can prevent your symptoms from affecting you as they did before.

Pregnancy Before Recovery

It is vital that you are fully recovered from an episode of postpartum depression before you attempt to get pregnant again. If you become pregnant again while you are still symptomatic from a previous PPD, or within the first year after giving birth, you risk exacerbating your illness. Every pregnancy is different and presents a new set of challenges. If you are still grappling with PPD, you may not yet be mentally equipped to deal with another pregnancy and postpartum period. You have a 50 percent chance of developing postpartum depression again with future pregnancies if you've fully recovered from a previous episode. If you haven't recovered, another postpartum depression will be very difficult to avoid, and could potentially be a lot worse. PPD sufferer Eliza S. got pregnant again when her son was only six months old and she was not fully recovered from her PPD. A short time later she had a miscarriage, which devastated her and forced her to start her recovery from postpartum depression all over again. This time, though, she felt twice as bad.

> *"I learned the hard way that what I was told (wait at least a year to become pregnant) was very good advice."*
> —Eliza S.

Unusual Circumstances

There are certain situations, which we call "unusual circumstances," that can make you more susceptible to postpartum depression. Having an abortion, miscarriage, interrupted pregnancy, or a stillbirth can be very traumatic and put you at greater risk for PPD. Women who have fertility problems, or have a partner with a fertility problem, and need an egg or sperm donation in order to have a child are at greater risk. So are women who need to use a surrogate mother. Women who are having multiples and must use the process of **reduction** to safeguard the health of their babies or because of financial strain are at greater risk. Women who have unexpected multiple births, meaning they don't find out they are having more than one baby until delivery, are at increased risk. So are those who have given a child up for adoption in the past. Women with a history of alcohol or drug abuse are at increased risk as well, because addiction causes personality changes and compromises the integrity and well-being of the body and mind. Addiction also indicates some sort of maladaption in life that makes women more susceptible to PPD.

Psychological Risk Factors

Personality

There are certain personality types that are vulnerable to PPD. The perfectionist woman with unrealistic expectations and anticipations is at risk. If you expect yourself to get everything right while learning how to take care of your child, you're setting yourself up for failure. Every new mom makes mistakes, but those who punish themselves excessively for making mistakes can chip away at their own self-esteem and develop postpartum problems, including postpartum depression.

Women with a strong need for control are also at risk. Having a baby will turn your life upside down, and your daily routine will change dramatically. You'll find that your baby has much of the control you once had. Your life now revolves around his schedule of eating and sleeping, and even that is often unpredictable. There's no controlling this, and it leads many women to feel frustrated and out of control.

Women who excessively worry or have obsessive-compulsive

tendencies are at risk for postpartum depression as well. Worrying too much is never a good thing, but when you're in the middle of a major life change like having a baby, it can be downright damaging. Many women focus their worry on their babies. They're concerned about every cough, every cry. They obsess about things that could happen to their baby, like car accidents or kidnappings. Other women focus their worry on themselves: Am I a good mother? Am I doing the right things? Will I ever lose my pregnancy weight? Will I ever feel like my old self again? The more you worry or think negatively about yourself or your baby, the more likely you are to have trouble adjusting to this life change you're going through.

Unwanted and Unplanned Pregnancy

Unwanted or unplanned pregnancies are typically considered single women's issues, but the truth is that many women in committed relationships or marriages also find themselves in these types of situations. Being pregnant when you don't want to be is extremely stressful. So is having an unplanned pregnancy. Some women with unplanned pregnancies accept their situation with time and come to embrace their pregnancy. But that is not always the case. Women who carry an unwanted child often feel resentment toward their baby and have difficulty developing the bond that most mothers are able to form with their unborn children. They are also often very critical of themselves for winding up in this situation. These factors can lead to depression both during pregnancy and postpartum.

Traumatic Birth Experience

Many women experience considerable pain and anxiety during labor and childbirth. For some, the stress of childbirth is so severe that it has lingering psychological effects afterward, or worse, they develop postpartum post-traumatic stress disorder. The emotional trauma of having to undergo an emergency C-section, or having the anesthesia ineffectively delivered during a C-section (causing you to feel pain during the procedure), are examples of traumatic birth experiences that could leave you vulnerable to PPD. So is delivering a premature baby. Women are usually unprepared for a premature birth and are very worried about their babies' health. They are also separated from their babies, making it difficult to breast-feed or to care for them.

Other traumatic experiences include:

- your baby going into distress during or after delivery
- having multiple births
- having an episiotomy
- enduring an especially long labor
- feeling as though you have no control over what's happening to your body during the birth
- the birth happening too quickly
- experiencing considerable postpartum pain, from C-section recovery or complications

Childhood Experiences

We are all influenced by how we grew up, by events from our childhood, and the birth of a baby tends to rekindle past crises. Women whose needs were not met during childhood, meaning they were not nurtured or given positive feedback, and women who grew up with an alcoholic parent are more susceptible to postpartum depression. So are women who suffered from sexual, physical, or emotional abuse as a child, especially if they haven't worked through their childhood issues properly.

While physical and sexual abuse are self-explanatory, emotional abuse can be more difficult to define, as it can take so many different forms. Emotional abuse involves being ridiculed, criticized, and treated disrespectfully. Emotional abuse often happens in families where one or both parents are alcoholics, drug addicts, or suffer from psychological illness. Children who are abused in any way often grow up with low self-esteem and a poor sense of identity. Caring for a newborn is a huge responsibility that challenges even the healthiest woman's self-esteem and sense of identity, so entering this situation with self-esteem and identity issues can make the postpartum period a very difficult time. Low self-esteem can make you question your ability to be a good mom. You may find that having a baby stirs up painful memories of what it was like for you to live in a dysfunctional household. All of this can cause you extreme anxiety and distress, and may ultimately lead to postpartum depression.

A difficult relationship with your mother is also a risk factor for PPD. Every mother-daughter relationship has its rough times, but the rockier your relationship, the greater your risk for having postpartum difficulties. Being separated from a parent during childhood (either through death or divorce) is also a risk factor, and if your mother is deceased, you are especially susceptible to postpartum depression.

Recent Stressful Life Events

The more stressful events you experience during your pregnancy and postpartum period, the greater your odds are for developing postpartum depression. Pregnancy, childbirth, and the early postpartum period are considered stressful life events themselves, so additional stress can sometimes be enough to push you over the edge. Stressful life events include the death or serious illness of a loved one, a change in your finances, changing or losing a job, relocating to a new town, or even moving into a new home in the same town you live in now. Many women also feel very anxious about the thought of returning to work after their maternity leave. The stress of having to find child care for their baby and the mixed emotions many women feel about leaving their baby in someone else's care can have a significant effect on their emotional well-being during the postpartum period.

Some stressful life events are out of your control, but for those you can choose, such as buying a new house or changing jobs, it's better to wait until you've adjusted to the birth of your new baby. Now is the time to simplify your life, not complicate it. Focus on reducing your current stressors and learning relaxation techniques to help you through stressful moments. Being a new mother is tough, both physically and emotionally, and this will serve you well as you learn to adjust.

Difficulty Adapting to Change

As you read earlier, research shows that certain personality types are more susceptible to postpartum depression. The same is true for women with certain emotional traits, such as poor coping and adaptation skills. As you're well aware, having a baby is a huge life change, and it's stressful for every woman. But women who are able to look at the upheaval in a positive way, who can roll with the punches and not be too self-critical when things go wrong, are better able to adapt to and cope with the changes a baby brings. If you're set in your ways and have difficulty accepting change, the postpartum period will be more difficult for you.

Colicky Baby

All newborns cry and are fussy to some degree, but infants who cry for three hours or more per day at least three days a week and are otherwise healthy have a condition called colic. No one's sure what causes colic—researchers theorize it could be anything from stomach pain to the baby's temperament. Colic usually begins three to six weeks after birth and can last until the baby reaches three months old. Coping with a colicky baby is one of the more difficult jobs on earth, and it puts an enormous strain on a mother's relationship with her baby. It's very hard to remain positive when your baby cries for extended periods of time and you can't find a way to console him. Women with colicky babies often become extremely fatigued and anxious and are prone to postpartum depression, in part because they feel like failures for not being able to soothe their babies.

It's easy to see how mothers of colicky babies might become depressed, but it wasn't until a study published by Pamela High, MD, a Brown Medical School professor, and a group of Rhode Island Department of Health family health experts in May 2006 that there was a definitive link proven between depression and colic. In the study, mothers who reported depression were more than twice as likely to report infant inconsolability, and women with inconsolable babies were more than two times as likely to report depression. The study makes it clear that depression and inconsolable babies are strong predictors of each other.

Unhappiness with Baby's Gender

When asked whether they want a boy or a girl, most pregnant women will say that they don't care what the sex of their baby is, as long as the baby is healthy. But the truth is that many of us have our hearts set on having the boy or the girl we've been dreaming about, and when that doesn't happen, it can be a big letdown. Women who are disappointed by the gender of their babies usually feel very guilty about feeling this way, and that guilt can put them at greater risk for postpartum depression.

> *"I spent all my life dreaming about Barbie dolls and pink dresses. I was really despondent to learn I was having a boy. I don't like baseball."*
>
> —Diane O.

This isn't just a problem for women. Your partner may be the one who has his heart set on the gender of your baby, and if, for example, you give birth to a girl instead of a boy and you sense your partner is disappointed, you may feel enormous guilt about not giving him what he so badly wanted.

Excessive Weight Gain

Women who put on an excessive amount of weight during their pregnancy, in the neighborhood of fifty pounds or more, are at greater risk for PPD. There are two main reasons for this.

First, being overweight puts a strain on you physically and makes pregnancy and the postpartum period more difficult. Excessive weight gain during pregnancy makes you more susceptible to gestational diabetes, which can cause complications for you and your baby. Carrying a lot of extra weight will also make it more difficult for you to recover from childbirth and keep up with the demands of your newborn. Overweight women have less energy than women within the normal weight range, and energy is something you desperately need during your postpartum period.

Second, being overweight can have a negative psychological effect on you. It takes months to lose baby weight, even when you gain just a normal amount, and that's hard on every woman's psyche. But if you've gained a lot of extra weight, it could take much longer than a few months for you to return to your pre-pregnancy form, and this can be very discouraging and depressing. Women who have struggled with self-esteem issues in the past may be hit especially hard by excessive weight gain, because they often find it more difficult to handle not looking their best.

Feeling Less Attractive

Pregnancy creates profound changes in your body, and not all of them disappear once the baby is born. It takes many women months (even years) to lose the extra weight they gained during their pregnancy. Even after you lose the weight, the shape of your body can change permanently, and your clothes won't necessarily fit you the same way. Taking care of a baby often leaves you with little or no time to take care of yourself. Showers can be few and far between. You may not be able to make it to the hairdresser, so your hair looks shaggy and your highlights have grown out. You may not have figured out a way to get that much-needed eyebrow wax since you had the baby. There are a million little things that we do to make ourselves feel attractive that we can't find the time or energy for in the months after the baby comes. Then we look in the mirror and don't like what we see, but don't know what to do about it. Feeling less attractive is a definite risk factor for PPD.

Social Risk Factors

Culture Shock

Regardless of your circumstances, having a new baby requires you to make a complete change in your lifestyle. But that lifestyle change seems to be the most profound for career-oriented women who are making a radical move from full-time professional career to full-time motherhood. (This applies to women who are on maternity leave as well, because they are full-time mothers for at least a few months.) These women often have a very difficult time adjusting to their new life. At their job, they knew what to do and how to do it, and their work usually gave them some degree of self-satisfaction. They could take breaks when they needed them and have adult interaction whenever they wanted. Motherhood is a totally different ballpark. Now they don't know how to do anything. They feel overwhelmed and unsure of themselves. They are working longer, harder hours, but they are not getting paid and don't feel as productive. They have hardly any adult interaction and spend the majority of their days trying to figure out how to understand and meet their baby's needs. Talk about culture shock! It's easy to see how a radical lifestyle change like this could help spark postpartum depression.

Relationship Problems

One of the highest predictors for postpartum depression is the stability of your relationship with your partner. Any problems you may have had with your partner before or during your pregnancy, such as communication issues, intimacy issues, or difficulty making enough time for each other, will only worsen after the birth. You're already under an enormous amount of stress, so if you perceive your partner as being unsupportive or unavailable in some way, it can be devastating. Taking care of a newborn and adjusting to life with a child puts strain on even the strongest relationships, and shaky relationships are in danger of unraveling during the postpartum period. If you are pregnant or thinking about getting pregnant and are having relationship difficulties, seek professional counseling now. Your relationship with your partner is crucial to your family's harmony, and you must do everything you can to maintain a strong, loving bond. If you are in the throes of PPD now, address your postpartum depression first and then seek out couples counseling. You can't take care of everything at the same time, and your health and well-being must come first.

Weak Support System

You have a greater chance of experiencing postpartum depression if you lack a strong support system of family and friends, or if you have no family living near you. Your support system is made up of the people in your life who are there to help you through the tough times with the baby. A strong support system is crucial to your recovery after your baby is born. You need to be able to talk with people you trust and who care about you and what you're going through. Not only is it a relief to share your feelings and frustrations with others, but it can also help you see that you're not alone in your struggles. Every woman has to find her way through the postpartum period, and when you open up about your difficulties, you'll learn how other women coped successfully with those same issues. You'll gain a sense of hope and acceptance that will buoy you through future tough times.

A good support system will also be there to provide physical support, such as babysitting and helping around the house. The people in your support system will help you create opportunities to get the rest and time you need to make a speedy postpartum recovery.

The weaker your support system, the more susceptible you are to postpartum depression. You need opportunities to take care of yourself, to replenish your emotional and physical resources after childbirth. If you don't have people you can lean on, who will listen and offer advice when you need to talk or watch the baby for a few hours while you take a break, it will take you longer to recover from the birth and leave you vulnerable to depression.

Being a Single Mother

Another risk factor for PPD is the stress associated with being a single mother. Single moms are often strapped with the burden of working full-time (or even more than one job) to financially support their child, doing all the housework and taking care of all of their child's needs with no help from a partner. They have an even larger than normal amount of responsibility to carry on their shoulders, and it's not hard to see how this can lead to increased stress and emotional issues. Single moms are especially at risk if they don't have a good support system to rely on for help with caring for their baby. (Single women who find they are having an unplanned or unwanted pregnancy are also at even greater risk. See page 63 for more information.)

Teenagers make up a large portion of the single mothers in the United States, and they are at even greater risk for postpartum difficulties. In the vast majority of cases, teen pregnancies are unplanned, which can make the adjustment to motherhood even harder than normal. (This is true for women of any age, not just teenage mothers.) They are usually not emotionally prepared for motherhood, as they often still feel like children themselves. They may need to drop out of school to take care of their baby, which can damage their potential for future success in the workplace and isolate them even further. Some teenage mothers continue to live at home so that their parents can help them. If their relationship with their parents is good, having that built-in support system is a great thing. But sadly, many women with troubled family relationships find that living at home with a new baby only exacerbates the family problems they've already been experiencing.

Regardless of your age, as a single mother you need all the help you can get during your postpartum period. Now is the time to call on your family and friends to lend a hand while you get back on your feet. If you don't have a support system you can depend on, look for help in your community. Many churches have programs where you can drop off your baby for a few hours or have someone visit your home to help out. Your local YMCA may also offer babysitting on the weekends or day care while you're at work.

Maternal Age

It's not uncommon for older moms to run into problems both during their pregnancies and postpartum, which can contribute to

PPD. Older moms are more likely to develop health problems, have more physical risk factors than younger moms, and often have less energy, less patience, and less ability to cope with the tremendous changes that occur in their bodies and lives. As we've mentioned repeatedly, having a baby is a *huge* life change, and older women, who are often set in their ways, can find it very difficult to adapt. Having a baby later in life is also more disruptive to their relationships with their partners than it usually is for younger moms, because older couples are more set in their ways. Late-in-life babies can also cause big changes to an older couple's life plan. For instance, your partner may not be able to retire when he had planned because of the expense of supporting a new baby. This can cause serious relationship friction.

Unemployment or Financial Problems

It's important to be financially secure when you start your family. If you are pregnant or have just had your baby and are worried that you or your partner are not earning enough money to support your family, that's a huge stressor in your life. Money is the number one issue couples argue about, and if there isn't enough to meet your family's needs, it's even easier to feel angry and depressed over your situation.

If you or your partner become unemployed, that's also a risk factor for PPD. You're now faced with a dramatically lower or nonexistent income, and that's scary. The job market is tough these days, and getting a new job can often take months. You or your partner may have to take a salary cut or even relocate in order to secure a new job. Day after day of worrying about money issues and job prospects on top of taking care of your baby will wear you out emotionally, and can lead to depression.

Having financial problems can also prevent you from hiring help around the house or with the baby when you need it. Money problems may also stop you from getting certain types of medical help that you may need that aren't covered by your insurance policy. For instance, some insurance companies don't cover therapy, or they cover only a certain (usually insufficient) number of sessions (see pages 106–108 in chapter 5 for more information).

Fertility Treatments

There are many psychological factors surrounding fertility treatment, all of which can have an impact on your emotional state and contribute to PPD.

Many women feel ashamed and embarrassed when they cannot conceive a child naturally. They consider themselves failures and feel that they can't do anything right.

> *"If having a baby is supposed to be so natural, why didn't someone tell my body that? I felt inadequate. I wanted to give my husband a baby and I couldn't do it by myself. I felt like a failure."*
>
> —Kristen B.

The stress of simply going through fertility treatments is enormous. There are several different types of treatments—from in vitro fertilization (IVF) to drug programs to surgery—and some of these treatments can be long and even physically painful. Some of the infertility medications that are given, such as Clomid, can produce PPD-like symptoms. If the treatment is unsuccessful, it can be incredibly disheartening for you and your partner. Statistics show that it may very well take repeated treatments in order for you to conceive, and fertility treatments are expensive. They can result in a serious financial strain, which can create new problems in your relationship with your partner.

Short Hospital Stays

The length of time women stay in the hospital after giving birth has decreased significantly over the last several decades, in large part because of the insurance industry's reluctance to cover more than a few days. Today, women who have a normal vaginal delivery are hospitalized for just twenty-four to forty-eight hours, as opposed to four days back in the 1970s. Today, the typical hospital stay for women who've had C-sections ranges from forty-eight to seventy-two hours, though some hospitals will keep you for as long as ninety-six hours. In the 1970s, women were hospitalized for approximately eight days for C-section deliveries. For many women, such short hospital stays are simply not enough time to recover from the birth and adjust to having a baby. Many moms need to be cared for longer and feel completely unprepared to leave, and the transition to home can be very difficult for them.

Case Mismanagement

Another risk factor for PPD is something we call case mismanagement. Case mismanagement refers to a situation where, for instance, you had antepartum depression and you were misdiagnosed or improperly treated for it. You could have been given improper medication or no medication at all when you clearly would have benefited from it. Case mismanagement also refers to a situation where you were given wrong information about antepartum depression or postpartum depression, or given no information at all.

Exhaustion from Caring for a New Baby and Other Siblings

It's extremely difficult to adjust to a new baby in the house, not just for you but for your partner and your other children as well. Now you must figure out a way to meet the needs of your other kids and help them through this adjustment period. This is extremely tough work. With a new baby in the house, it's easy for your expectations of your older children to become unrealistic, and it can therefore become exhausting when they don't live up to them. New moms have a tendency to have a shorter fuse with their older children, because they can't get mad at the baby. This is a natural phenomenon, and you should be aware of it. You need to keep in mind that your behavioral expectations for your older kids must be age-related and realistic. Expecting more from them than they are developmentally able to give will create a bad dynamic and a lot of unnecessary frustration. You also need to cut yourself some slack. No matter what their ages, your children are continually growing and changing. Their personalities are still forming. This means you are still learning how to parent, but you are now dealing with two or more different developmental stages at the same time. This is stressful and exhausting and puts you at greater risk for developing PPD.

Ways to Reduce Your Risk for Developing PPD

Although there's no proven way to avoid developing postpartum depression, there are steps you can take to protect yourself and reduce your risk. First of all, you should be proactive and find out if you are at risk. In addition to scrutinizing the risk factors we describe in this chapter, set up an appointment with a qualified health-care professional to discuss your situation. He or she can help you minimize any risk factors within your control and help you come up with a plan to deal with PPD if it does occur. Diane G. was evaluated before getting pregnant, because she gave up a baby for adoption at age sixteen and felt that she needed to resolve her past in order to move forward. She has three kids now and did not develop postpartum depression after any of the births.

Here are some more tips for reducing your risk:

Educate yourself. Learn everything you can about postpartum depression. This will enable you to recognize the condition if it occurs and get help for it quickly. You will also be able to give your health-care practitioners the information they need to help you recover.

Sleep and eat appropriately. A nutritious diet and a sufficient amount of sleep are critical to your health and well-being. Do your best to eat right and get as much sleep as you can, both during your pregnancy and your postpartum period. (See chapter 6 for advice on proper sleep and nutrition.)

Exercise. Exercise is a key component in reducing your risk for PPD. Squeezing in even fifteen minutes of walking a day will elevate your mood and help you feel better about and in more control of your body. (See chapter 6 for advice on exercise.)

Avoid making major life changes during or right after childbirth. If at all possible, don't make any big life decisions, such as buying a house or changing jobs, during or right after your pregnancy. Keeping your life as simple and stress-free as possible will make your postpartum recovery faster and easier.

Let your feelings be known in the delivery room. Don't be afraid to speak up and express your needs and wants in the delivery room. It's important that your delivery be as comfortable as possible. If you want an epidural, tell the attending physicians. If you're uncomfortable, tell them.

Enlist good support during birthing. Make sure to surround yourself with people who can give you the support you need during childbirth. Perhaps that's your partner, or maybe it's your mother, your partner, and your best friend. You should also consider hiring a **doula** to help you through the process (see chapter 7 for more information). Do whatever it takes to feel supported during delivery in order to have the best possible experience.

Prepare yourself well for childbirth. Taking a childbirth education class is helpful, but don't stop there. Read as many books or articles on the topic as you can manage. Talk to other women about their experiences. Many childbirth classes skim over crucial aspects of childbirth, like C-sections, and you should be well informed on every possible outcome in the delivery room so that there will be no surprises. If you know what to expect, you're less apt to have a traumatic childbirth experience.

Enlist household help during the postpartum period. You will be in no condition to cook meals and clean the house in the first few weeks after your baby is born, especially if you have a C-section, so arrange for people in your support system to help you. Have someone go grocery shopping for you to stock up on frozen entrees and easy snacks. Let your sister vacuum the living room floor for you. Your support system is there to help—use them. If you don't have a support system you can depend on, think about hiring outside help until you're back on your feet. Having someone come to your house to clean up twice a week and even cook some meals for your family will be a huge relief for you.

Find strong emotional support—and take advantage of it. Your support system is also there for you to lean on when you're feeling frustrated, overwhelmed, or just plain tired. Talk to them about how you're feeling and how your life is changing. You'll feel a lot better after you've vented. You should also use your support system to create some time for yourself whenever you can. Let your mother watch the baby while you take a long, hot bath. Let your best friend babysit while you and your partner go out for dinner.

Attend a PPD support group. The best support often comes from people who have been where you are and know what you are going through. Talk to your obstetrician, a therapist, your baby's pediatrician, or other moms, and find out where your local PPD support group meets.

FOUR

How Is
Postpartum
Depression Diagnosed?

THE FIRST STEP in the diagnosis process is to make the decision to seek help. A key part of recovering from postpartum depression is recognizing and accepting that you have this condition and taking control of your health. Having postpartum depression does not make you a defective person, a bad mother, or flawed. Hundreds of thousands of women go through the same experience every year, even though they don't often tell people. With the right help, you can overcome PPD and be happy again.

Roadblocks to Diagnosis

Getting diagnosed with postpartum depression isn't always easy. One of the biggest problems women run into when they reach out for help is that their health-care practitioners underestimate what they're going through. Many women are told that they have the baby blues and that it will soon go away on its own when they're really suffering from the more serious postpartum depression. Many physicians simply don't know enough about PPD to recognize the condition or make the proper diagnosis. Remember this: you are the expert on how you're feeling, and now is the time to trust your instincts—if you feel like something is wrong, then something is wrong. It's as simple as that. If this happens to you, push the issue with your health professional. Explain that you've been feeling this way for over two weeks (anything less than two weeks *could* actually be the baby blues) and that you don't think what's going on is normal. It's a really good idea to fill out and bring in the Postpartum Depression Checklist on page 82 to show to your health professional. If she is still dismissive, make an appointment to see someone else (see page 84 for a list of health professionals who can help you). You can also talk with other moms or call the leader of a local support group to get a list of reputable health-care practitioners. Don't stop until you've found the help that you need and deserve.

In addition to dismissive health-care practitioners, there are several other reasons why postpartum depression isn't always detected as quickly as it should be:

Women aren't clear about what's "normal." The concept of the baby blues is common, and most women expect to have some kind of adjustment period after their baby is born. As you read in chapter 1, the baby blues and PPD share many of the same symptoms, and this makes it difficult for many first-time mothers to recognize that what they are experiencing is not within the norm and to reach out for help.

Women sabotage themselves by not being honest. Too many women don't want to talk about how they're feeling, because saying it out loud will make it real. They deny their feelings to themselves and to the people around them and pretend that they are happy, which is both exhausting and detrimental to their well-being. It's important for women to be honest about how they are feeling; otherwise they will suffer needlessly, because they may never be diagnosed, or receive improper treatment since their health-care practitioners aren't aware of the true nature or extent of their condition. They also won't receive the support they need at home, because their friends and family won't know they need it.

Societal pressures. Our society expects women to be "good mothers," so if a woman does recognize that something is wrong, she may be afraid or ashamed to admit it.

Fear of repercussions. Women with postpartum depression frequently think they are "going crazy" and worry that if they share these thoughts with a health-care professional, they will be "locked up" or someone will take their baby away from them. Liz A. was afraid to tell her midwife about her feelings. When Liz finally told her that she was afraid to be alone with her baby, her midwife called 911 and had Liz taken away on a stretcher to a mental health crisis center in front of her other daughter and her husband, because, as the midwife said, "We don't want another Andrea Yates on our hands." This kind of response is why women are so afraid to admit to their feelings.

Women don't know where to get help. Another complicating factor is that women are often confused about whom to turn to. They may not be scheduled to see their gynecologist for another year, and they think of their child's pediatrician as being focused on the child, not as someone they could turn to for help. As you'll learn in this chapter, there are several types of health-care practitioners who can help you, but you do need to be careful who you see. Make sure you make an appointment with an experienced PPD expert (see pages 84–85 later in this chapter for more information).

Insurance companies. These days health-care practitioners are under immense pressure from insurance companies to evaluate more patients in less time, so psychological issues like postpartum depression are frequently given little attention from even the most thoughtful clinicians. (See pages 106–108 in chapter 5 for more information.)

When to Seek Help

Providing that you aren't having thoughts of harming yourself or others, hallucinations, or delusional thoughts, you can wait up to two weeks to see whether your depressive symptoms will go away. After that point, however, it's important to see your health-care practitioner. The earlier you are treated, the more quickly you will recover, and the less your baby's development will be affected by your condition. You should also seek help any time you feel your symptoms are intolerable. For instance, if you are having debilitating panic attacks, don't suffer through them for two weeks before calling your health-care practitioner for help. Call right now for an appointment.

IN CASE OF EMERGENCY

IF YOU are afraid you cannot keep from harming yourself, your baby, or another person, call 911 or other emergency services. You can also call the national suicide hotline, known as the National Hopeline Network, at 1-800-784-2433, or the National Child Abuse Hotline at 1-800-422-4453.

Joyce has created the Postpartum Depression Checklist, which we provide below, to help her patients track their postpartum depression symptoms over the span of two weeks. This helps both Joyce and her patients understand how PPD is affecting them and enables her to treat them accordingly. We strongly suggest that you fill it out and bring it with you to your first appointment.

POSTPARTUM DEPRESSION CHECKLIST

THIS CHECKLIST can be used as early as two weeks postpartum.
It is intended to help you identify your postpartum symptoms. It is not a substitute for a professional medical evaluation.
Rate your level of discomfort each day for 10 days, using a scale of 0 to 10.
0 being Not at All and 10 being the Most Severe

SYMPTOMS	DAY									
	1	2	3	4	5	6	7	8	9	10
Anger										
Anxiety attacks										
Appetite, increase or loss of										
Conflicts/personal relationships										
Crying spells										
Decreased interest in appearance										
Decreased motivation										
Depression										
Fatigue										
Fear of harming yourself/others*										
Fear that you will harm baby*										
Fearfulness										
Feeling too good										
Feelings of guilt										
Feelings of panic										
Feeling others are not supportive										
Feeling no love for baby										
Forgetfulness										
Frustration										
Hopelessness										
Insomnia										

SYMPTOMS	DAY									
	1	2	3	4	5	6	7	8	9	10
Irritability										
Loss of sexual desire										
Low self-esteem										
Mental confusion										
Mood swings										
Obsessive, repetitive thoughts*										
Panic										
Poor ability to concentrate										
Suicidal thoughts*										
Weight gain/loss										

*Seek immediate professional help

Finding the Right Health Professional

An **obstetrician** is usually the first health professional women see after giving birth, as most of them require you to come in for a medical check four to eight weeks after childbirth. This is a great time to share what you're feeling with your health-care practitioner. She may ask you point blank if you're feeling sad or anxious. Tell the truth. You may not want to admit what's going on to your friends and family yet, but your health-care practitioner is only there to help you.

If your follow-up obstetrician appointment has come and gone, or if your obstetrician didn't ask and you didn't tell her about your PPD symptoms, then you need to choose which health-care practitioner you're going to see. You could make another appointment with your obstetrician, but there are several other kinds of health professionals who are qualified to diagnose and manage your recovery from postpartum depression as well. The most important thing is for you to choose someone with whom you feel comfortable. Here's a list of health-care providers who can help you:

General practitioner. General practitioners are medical doctors who diagnose and treat most types of health conditions or diseases and do not specialize in any particular area of medicine. They provide basic medical service for people of all age groups and both genders.

Family doctor. Family medicine physicians, also called family practice physicians, are medical doctors who specialize in the total health care of the individual and the family. They can diagnose and treat a variety of health conditions and diseases for people of all ages and both genders. Some family doctors often further specialize in another area of medicine, such as the care of older adults (geriatric medicine) or people who have sports injuries (sports medicine).

Psychiatrist. Psychiatrists are medical doctors who specialize in the diagnosis and treatment of mental health problems, such as depression. They provide counseling and are licensed to prescribe medications to treat mental illness.

Physician assistant. Physician assistants (PAs) are health professionals who practice medicine under a doctor's supervision in medical and surgical settings. They can perform routine examinations, order laboratory work and X-rays, prescribe medications, and counsel people about their health.

Nurse practitioner. Nurse practitioners (NPs) are registered nurses (RNs) who have advanced education and clinical training. They can perform physical examinations, diagnose and treat health problems, order lab work and X-rays, prescribe medications, and provide health information.

What to Look for in a Health Professional

While all of the above-mentioned health professionals can treat your condition, it's best to find someone who has experience treating postpartum depression. If none of your current health-care practitioners fits the bill, ask if they can refer you to a colleague who's experienced with PPD. If your current health-care practitioners can't help you, here are some other good ways to find a qualified professional:

- Speak to the leader of your local PPD support group—she can certainly refer you to a good PPD specialist in your area.
- Every state is supposed to provide a toll-free phone number to help its residents locate support groups. If you don't have a local PPD support group, look in your Yellow Pages for your state's 800 number and call to find out where the closest one meets. Then call the leader of that group and ask her to recommend a good health-care practitioner.
- Call your insurance company and get a referral for someone they feel is qualified.
- Call Postpartum Support International at 800-944-4773—they have listings for PPD specialists all over the country.
- Ask other moms who have recently had babies.

Once you've made an appointment with a recommended health-care practitioner, you need to get prepared for your first visit. As we mentioned earlier in this chapter, it's a very good idea for you to fill out and bring the Postpartum Depression Checklist from page 82 to your appointment. This checklist will help you give your health-care practitioner the information she needs to properly diagnose and treat you. You should also prepare a list of questions to ask so that you can assess her experience and abilities and decide whether you think you will be comfortable under her care. Here are some questions we encourage you to ask:

- Are you familiar with ante- and postpartum disorders?
- What has been your experience with them?
- How many patients have you treated with ante- and postpartum depression?
- Are you up-to-date on the most recent research?
- Do you have current material for me to read?

- In your practice, do you use the Edinburgh Postnatal Depression Scale? (We provide the Edinburgh Postnatal Depression Scale on page 89.)
- Do you have patients I can speak with who have had PPD?
- Do you provide resources so that I can get more information on PPD?
- Do you know of a support group I can attend?
- What are your feelings about PPD? Do you consider it a real medical illness?

Exams and Tests

There are no laboratory tests available to definitively diagnose postpartum depression, so your health-care practitioner will have to perform a comprehensive evaluation to arrive at a diagnosis.

Ruling Out Other Conditions

The first thing your health-care practitioner will do is run tests to rule out any other medical conditions that may be causing or exacerbating your symptoms, such as:

Postpartum thyroiditis. Postpartum thyroiditis is a condition in which the thyroid becomes inflamed and dysfunctional after delivery, because of antibodies. Antithyroid antibodies circulate in the body, causing either too much or too little thyroid hormone to be released. Too much thyroid hormone will cause you to have an overactive thyroid gland, while too little will result in an underactive thyroid.

Postpartum thyroiditis typically follows a pattern: at first you become hyperthyroid and might feel breathless, nervous, mentally confused, have unexplained weight loss, or trouble sleeping. This phase usually appears anytime between one and four months after the birth of the baby.

In the second phase, which usually shows up three to eight

months postpartum, the body's hormones are again out of whack. Instead of releasing too much thyroid hormone, the body releases too little, and you become hypothyroid. Symptoms of this stage might be depression, fatigue, weight gain or difficulty losing weight, and an enlarged thyroid gland or sensation of pressure in your neck.

Postpartum thyroiditis occurs in 5 to 10 percent of all pregnancies and can be easily detected and treated by your health professional. She will draw blood and have it tested to determine if a thyroid condition is causing your symptoms. If the results indicate a problem, she'll prescribe medication to restore your thyroid levels, and your symptoms will disappear.

Iron-deficiency anemia. Iron-deficiency anemia is a condition where a lack of iron decreases the number of red cells in your blood and prevents your organs from getting the proper amount of oxygen. It can cause you to feel weak, fatigued, and irritable. Pregnant women have a higher risk of developing anemia, because the demands of pregnancy on the body can deplete its iron stores. Anemia can also occur if you lost a significant amount of blood during delivery. A simple blood test can verify the presence of anemia, and treatment is often as easy as taking an iron supplement.

Gestational diabetes. Between 2 and 7 percent of women develop gestational diabetes during pregnancy. Pregnancy makes it more difficult for your body to use insulin to convert the glucose you get from food into energy, so your pancreas has to produce more insulin to do the job. Gestational diabetes happens when your pancreas can't keep up with your body's demand for insulin and your blood glucose levels become too high. Symptoms of gestational diabetes include weight gain, fatigue, and irritability. The condition usually disappears after childbirth, but it's not uncommon for it to linger for several weeks to a few months, and in rare cases it becomes a permanent condition.

Medication side effects. Several medications, such as some birth control pills, **metoclopramides** (a class of antinausea medication that is prescribed for pregnant women), and **carbamazepines** (a class of medication that controls seizures and relieves certain types of pain) can cause depression. Make sure to tell your health-care practitioner about every medication you've taken in the last year.

After ruling out these possibilities, you can expect your health-care practitioner to ask you some questions that will help her to accurately assess your symptoms and mental state.

The Interview

Your health-care practitioner needs to talk with you about your symptoms before coming to a conclusion about your diagnosis. This can be difficult, especially if you have not yet told anyone how you're feeling, but it's crucial that you tell your health-care practitioner everything that you've been experiencing. Don't hold anything back, especially if you've had thoughts about harming yourself or your baby. Remember, this is a *temporary* condition, and these hardest-to-talk-about symptoms are part of that condition, and they will disappear with proper treatment.

During this "interview," your health-care practitioner will ask you what your symptoms are, how bad they are, and how long they have lasted. This is where the Postpartum Depression Checklist comes in handy. It will help you remember all of your symptoms so you won't forget to mention any of them. She will ask whether you have ever had similar symptoms before. You will also be asked about your risk factors for depression, such as family or marital problems, other stresses, mental illness in family members, and drug and alcohol use (see chapter 3 for more information on risk factors).

In addition to the checklist and your list of questions for the health-care practitioner, it's a good idea for you to jot down any thoughts or concerns you have about your condition or your symptoms. You can never give your health-care practitioner too much information. It's also wise to bring your partner, a family member, or some other support person with you for your first appointment. You're likely very upset right now, and you may forget much of what your health-care practitioner will tell you. If this happens, your support person will be able to answer questions about the appointment for you when you get home.

Health-care practitioners generally will diagnose and recommend treatment for postpartum depression if you've had five or more of the following symptoms (including the first or second) for most of each day over the past two weeks.

- depressed mood—tearfulness, hopelessness, and feeling empty inside, with or without severe anxiety
- loss of pleasure in either all or almost all of your daily activities
- appetite and weight change—usually a drop in appetite and weight, but sometimes the opposite
- sleep problems—usually trouble with sleeping, even when your baby is sleeping
- noticeable change in how you walk and talk—you may seem restless or move very slowly
- extreme fatigue or loss of energy
- feelings of worthlessness or guilt, with no reasonable cause
- difficulty concentrating and making decisions
- thoughts about death or suicide

Your health-care practitioner will also likely ask you to take one or both of these two screening tests created to detect PPD: the Edinburgh Postnatal Depression Scale and the Postpartum Depression Screening Scale.

The Edinburgh Postnatal Depression Scale (EDPS)

The EPDS was developed in 1987 at health centers in Livingston and Edinburgh, Scotland, to assist primary-care health professionals in detecting postpartum depression in new mothers. Since that time, the scale has been validated, and evidence from a number of research studies has confirmed the tool to be both reliable and sensitive in detecting depression. To complete the test, underline the response that comes closest to how you have been feeling in the past seven days.

1. I have been able to laugh and see the funny side of things.
   A. As much as I always could
   B. Not quite so much now
   C. Definitely not so much now
   D. Not at all
2. I have looked forward with enjoyment to things.
   A. As much as I ever did
   B. Rather less than I used to
   C. Definitely less than I used to
   D. Hardly at all
3. I have blamed myself unnecessarily when things went wrong.
   A. Yes, most of the time
   B. Yes, some of the time
   C. Not very often
   D. No, never
4. I have been anxious or worried for no good reason.
   A. No, not at all
   B. Hardly ever
   C. Yes, sometimes
   D. Yes, very often
5. I have felt scared or panicky for no good reason.
   A. Yes, quite a lot
   B. Yes, sometimes
   C. No, not much
   D. No, not at all
6. Things have been getting on top of me.
   A. Yes, most of the time I haven't been able to cope at all
   B. Yes, sometimes I haven't been coping as well as usual
   C. No, most of the time I have coped quite well
   D. No, I have been coping as well as ever
7. I have been so unhappy that I have had difficulty sleeping.

A. Yes, most of the time
B. Yes, sometimes
C. Not very often
D. No, not at all

8. I have felt sad or miserable.
   A. Yes, most of the time
   B. Yes, quite often
   C. Not very often
   D. No, not at all

9. I have been so unhappy that I have been crying.
   A. Yes, most of the time
   B. Yes, quite often
   C. Only occasionally
   D. No, never

10. The thought of harming myself has occurred to me.
    A. Yes, quite often
    B. Sometimes
    C. Hardly ever
    D. Never

Source: J. L. Cox, J. M. Holden, R. Sagovsky, "Detection of postnatal depression: Development of the 10-item Edinburgh Postnatal Depression Scale," *British Journal of Psychiatry* 150 (June 1987), 782–86.

CALCULATING YOUR SCORE

Your responses are scored 0, 1, 2, and 3 according to increased severity of the symptom. Your total score is calculated by adding together the scores for each of the ten items.

1. A=0, B=1, C=2, D=3
2. A=0, B=1, C=2, D=3
3. A=3, B=2, C=1, D=0
4. A=0, B=1, C=2, D=3
5. A=3, B=2, C=1, D=0
6. A=3, B=2, C=1, D=0
7. A=3, B=2, C=1, D=0

8. A=3, B=2, C=1, D=0
9. A=3, B=2, C=1, D=0
10. A=3, B=2, C=1, D=0

0–8 points:	low probability of depression
8–12 points:	most likely just dealing with life with a new baby or a case of baby blues
13–14 points:	signs leading to the possibility of PPD; take preventive measures
15+ points:	high probability of experiencing clinical postpartum depression

The Postpartum Depression Screening Scale (PDSS)

Developed by Cheryl Tatano Beck, DNSc, and Robert Gable, EdD, in 2000, the PDSS is a thirty-five-item questionnaire created specifically for postpartum women. The PDSS questions concern sleeping and eating disturbances, anxiety, insecurity, and emotional instability, feelings of guilt or shame, and suicidal thoughts. It's still considered relatively new and is not used as widely as the EPDS, but research has found that it has a greater specificity and sensitivity than the EPDS in screening for postpartum depression and is more likely to identify women with symptoms of sleep disturbance, mental confusion, and anxiety. Unlike the EDPS, which is free and easily obtainable on the Internet, you must either purchase access to the PDSS on the Internet or have a health-care practitioner administer it personally.

Other depression screening scales that can be used to assess the level of your depression include the Hamilton Rating Scale for Depression (HAM-D) and the Zung Self-Rating Scale. These are not used as frequently as the EDPS and the PDSS, however, because they were not created solely for postpartum women. In addition, the HAM-D was designed to measure the severity of illness in patients who have already been diagnosed with depression.

FIVE

Medications and Therapies

THE GOOD NEWS about postpartum depression is that it is a very treatable illness. Depending on the type and severity of your PPD, therapy alone could be enough to help you recover. But more often PPD treatment consists of a combination of medication and therapy. The general rule of thumb is that the longer you've been depressed and the more severe your symptoms, the more likely it is you will need medication to help you recover.

The Medications

Since postpartum depression is in part a problem with brain chemistry, it responds very well to medication. There are two categories of drugs that have proven effective for women with PPD: **antidepressants** (especially the SSRIs) and **antianxiety medications**. Your health-care practitioner may prescribe one specific drug for you, or a combination of drugs from each of the categories listed above.

It's important to say that taking medication is not an "easy fix." Since every woman's hormonal and chemical system is unique, medications affect different women in different ways. Sometimes it can take weeks of working with your health-care practitioner to find the right medication, the right dosage, or the right drug combination to help you. You may start to feel the beneficial effects of the medication within a few days, or it could take a few weeks. On the other hand, medication can be the fastest and most effective way to elevate your mood and allow you to begin to work through your postpartum issues. You should also note that medication alone, without therapy, is not considered a complete treatment for PPD. If you're on medication, you should also be in therapy. Medication will not fix the underlying reasons you developed postpartum depression in the first place, nor will it help you improve or cope with your risk factors.

Antidepressants

Antidepressants are the most frequently prescribed medication for women with postpartum depression. As we mentioned above, depression is caused in part by an imbalance of brain chemicals, specifically neurotransmitters called **norepinephrine** and **serotonin**. Antidepressant medications work by restoring the balance of these two chemicals in your brain. There are four categories of antidepressants that health-care practitioners prescribe: **tricyclics (TCAs), monoamine oxidase inhibitors (MAOIs), atypical antidepressants,** and **selective serotonergic reuptake inhibitors (SSRIs)**. A few things to keep in mind: It typically takes anywhere from one to three weeks for antidepressants to begin to work and for your symptoms to begin to improve. Every medication has side effects that you might experience, ranging from dry mouth and nausea to weight gain and loss of libido. Sometimes these side effects pass within a week, but you may need to switch medications one or more times to minimize your side effects, which can prolong the time it takes for you to feel better (see page 97 for tips on coping with side effects).

SELECTIVE SEROTONERGIC REUPTAKE INHIBITORS (SSRIs)

Today, a majority of women with postpartum depression are treated with selective serotonin reuptake inhibitors, which work by increasing the availability of the neurotransmitter serotonin in the brain. SSRIs differ from other antidepressants because they only affect your serotonin levels, leaving all other neurotransmitters unaffected. Studies suggest that they're just as effective as older-generation antidepressants, such as tricyclics and monoamine oxidase inhibitors, but have fewer side effects. That's not to say that SSRIs don't have side effects—research shows that they can cause nausea, headache, anxiety, dry mouth, insomnia, and a variety of sexual dysfunctions. But these side effects often pass quickly, and if not, are less bothersome than the side effects of other types of antidepressants. The three SSRIs that are most commonly prescribed for postpartum depression (with generic names in parentheses) are Prozac (fluoxetine), Zoloft (sertraline), and Paxil (paroxetine).

ATYPICAL ANTIDEPRESSANTS

Atypical antidepressants, the newest group of antidepressant, are so named because they don't fit well into any of the other antidepressant medication categories. Health-care practitioners often prescribe atypical antidepressants when other antidepressants have problematic side effects. For instance, sometimes certain selective serotonin reuptake inhibitors or other antidepressants can cause significant problems with sexual function. The atypical antidepressant Wellbutrin (bupropion) is less likely to cause sexual dysfunction than other antidepressants, though sometimes it can cause agitation. If you find you're having a sexual dysfunction side effect, like loss of libido or the inability to achieve orgasm, Wellbutrin may be prescribed instead of, or in addition to, an SSRI. Remeron (mirtazapine) may be useful if you are experiencing insomnia or agitation; however, it often causes weight gain. Desyrel (trazodone) is often used along with an SSRI to help with sleep disturbances. Four popular atypical antidepressants are Desyrel (trazodone), Effexor (venlafaxine), Remeron (mirtazapine), and Wellbutrin (bupropion).

TRICYCLICS (TCAs)

First used in the 1950s, tricyclics were the first line of treatment for depression until the 1980s, when SSRIs were created. Tricyclics are still used to treat severe depression, OCD, and panic disorder today, but not as frequently as SSRIs and atypical antidepressants. TCAs usually have the most significant side effects of any of the antidepressants, and are toxic in large doses, making accidental overdose (or intentional overdose if the woman has severe PPD and is feeling suicidal) a concern. Side effects include dry mouth, weight gain, constipation, blurred vision, **urinary retention**, and **orthostatic hypotension**, which is why many health-care practitioners avoid prescribing TCAs unless other antidepressants have proven ineffective. Here's a list of tricyclics that are frequently prescribed:

- Anafranil (clomipramine)
- Aventyl (nortriptyline)
- Elavil (amitriptyline)
- Ludiomil (maprotiline)
- Norpramin (desipramine)
- Pamelor (nortriptyline)
- Sinequan (doxepin)
- Surmontil (trimipramine)
- Tofranil-PM (imipramine pamoate)
- Vivactil (protriptyline)

MONOAMINE OXIDASE INHIBITORS (MAOIs)

Monoamine oxidase inhibitors affect the same neurotransmitters (serotonin and norepinephrine) that the tricyclics do, but they also affect the neurotransmitter **dopamine**. Monoamine oxidase inhibitors have not been widely tested and are not usually used to treat women with postpartum depression because of strict dietary constraints and the possible risk for a hypertensive crisis. MAOIs are never prescribed along with another drug because of the high risk for dangerous interactions. If you are taking an MAOI, you must stay away from foods with a high level of **tyramine**, such as many cheeses, pickled foods, chocolates, certain meats, beer, wine, and alcohol-free or reduced-alcohol beer and wine. The interaction of tyramine with MAOIs can cause a dangerously high increase in blood pressure, which can lead to a stroke. MAOIs can also cause a long list of side effects, such as drowsiness, nausea, diarrhea, fatigue, weight gain, and weakness. For these reasons health-care practitioners usually reserve MAOIs for women who don't respond to other antidepressant medications first.

As we mentioned earlier, MAOIs are not typically used for postpartum depression, but they can be very helpful for women who are suffering from atypical forms of major depression—people who are sensitive to rejection, who overeat and oversleep, and who react strongly to their environment. MAOIs reduce the sensitivity that leads these people to feel so easily hurt or rejected. Others who tend to respond very well to MAOIs are those who feel quite depressed but are able to surface from their depression from time to time and experience pleasure before plunging into depression again.

Three of the most commonly prescribed MAOIs are Nardil (phenelzine), Parnate (tranylcypromine), and Marplan (isocarboxazid).

COPING WITH MEDICATION SIDE EFFECTS

ANTIDEPRESSANTS CAN cause mild and usually temporary side effects in some people. This is because all medications have the potential for something called the **activation affect**, which is what happens when your body responds to a chemical when it first enters your system. Typically these effects are annoying but not serious. However, you should immediately tell your health-care practitioner about any unusual reactions or side effects that interfere with your ability to function. Following is a list of the most common side effects of antidepressants and tips for dealing with them:

- **Agitation (feeling jittery):** If this happens for the first time after the drug is taken (and isn't one of your PPD symptoms) and doesn't pass quickly, call your health-care practitioner. Or if agitation is a symptom you are experiencing because of your PPD and it worsens after you start on your medication, alert your health-care practitioner.
- **Bladder problems**: You may have infrequent trouble emptying your bladder, and the urine stream may not be as strong as usual; call your health-care practitioner if you have any pain.

- **Blurred vision**: This is infrequent and will pass soon. You don't need to get glasses.

- **Constipation**: Incorporate bran cereals, prunes, and plenty of fruit and vegetables into your diet, and drink lots of water. Exercise can also help.

- **Diarrhea**: Take Imodium. If it happens more than twice in one day, call your physician.

- **Dizziness**: Rising from your bed or a chair slowly will help.

- **Drowsiness as a daytime problem**: This usually passes soon, but until it does, don't drive or operate heavy equipment. The more sedating antidepressants are generally taken at bedtime to help sleep and minimize daytime drowsiness.

- **Dry mouth**: Drink lots of water; chew sugarless gum or sugarless candies; clean teeth daily.

- **Headache**: A headache you have as a side effect of an antidepressent will be unlike any headache you've ever experienced. Take Motrin or Tylenol. If it does not dissipate, alert your physician. These types of headaches usually go away quickly on their own.

- **Nausea**: When it occurs, it should do so only briefly. Try taking your medication with food. If that doesn't help or the nausea worsens, call your health-care practitioner.

- **Nervousness and insomnia (trouble falling asleep or waking often during the night)**: These may occur during the first few weeks; dosage reductions or time will usually resolve them. Try Benadryl for the insomnia, and be certain that you are taking the antidepressant in the morning unless otherwise directed by your physician.

- **Sexual problems**: Sexual functioning may change—you may experience loss of sex drive or ability to climax. Talk to your health-care practitioner about reducing your dosage or switching to a medication that has less possibility for sexual side effects, like Wellbutrin. Please note that loss of libido is common in postpartum women in general, not just in women with PPD.

Source: National Institute of Mental Health, *Depression,* Publication No. NIH99-3561 (1994; rev. 2000).

Antianxiety Medications

Antianxiety medications are designed to reduce anxiety and generally act to increase the neurotransmitter **GABA (gamma-aminobutyric acid),** which inhibits brain activity. In other words, GABA is the neurotransmitter that helps induce relaxation and sleep. There is one main category of antianxiety medications, called **benzodiazepines**. They are also referred to as **minor tranquilizers** and **anxiolytics**. Antianxiety medications are used to "take the edge off," or as a temporary Band-Aid to treat one or more PPD symptoms, not the whole illness. They are used to calm you and give you more clarity, not to sedate you.

Benzodiazepines

Benzodiazepines work to "quiet" different parts of your brain. Their major advantage is that they are fast-acting, as they take effect in a matter of minutes as opposed to days or weeks, like antidepressant medications do. Health-care practitioners often prescribe benzodiazepines for a few weeks or months to help women cope until their antidepressant medication kicks in, as well as for times of increased stress and hormonal fluctuations that may cause an increase in symptoms. They are especially effective in helping women suppress panic attacks. Benzodiazepines are also commonly used in conjunction with antidepressant medication to help with sleep, as some antidepressants can cause insomnia and benzodiazepines are useful in restoring your natural sleep-wake cycle. The main side effects of these minor tranquilizers are sedation and lightheadedness, but those conditions can usually be managed by adjusting the dosage you're taking.

Many women who are prescribed benzodiazepines are afraid they will become addicted to their medication. That's a valid concern, but since benzodiazepines are only used for a limited amount of time, the risk for addiction is considered quite low. Studies show that if addiction occurs, it occurs almost exclusively in women who have a history of abusing other drugs, such as alcohol, marijuana, or cocaine. In these cases, your health-care practitioner may prescribe Buspar (buspirone), which is the only benzodiazepine with no addiction potential. The downside to Buspar is that it has a delayed effectiveness similar to antidepressants, so you won't get immediate relief.

The most commonly prescribed benzodiazepines are Ativan (lorazepam), Klonopin (clonazepam), Xanax (alprazolam), and Buspar (buspirone).

Other Medications

There are two other drug categories that need mentioning: Antipsychotics and anti-mania medications, which are used to treat postpartum psychosis and postpartum mania, respectively, have been used to treat postpartum depression in certain instances. But these instances are very rare and are used only as a last resort for hard-to-treat cases where typical medications have failed.

Hormone Therapy

Using an estrogen patch—a patch containing estrogen that you wear on your skin—can help counteract the rapid drop in estrogen that accompanies childbirth. In a study of sixty-one women with postpartum depression, those who used the estrogen patch every day were less depressed than those who did not use it. However, estrogen therapy in the postpartum period may pose possible risks, such as decreased milk production, the risk of developing a blood clot in the legs that could travel to the lungs, and exacerbation of PPD symptoms. It's unlikely that hormone therapy will become a mainstream treatment for postpartum depression because of its risk factors and the limited amount of studies done thus far to prove its efficacy.

Electroconvulsive Therapy (ECT)

Many people think of electroconvulsive therapy as "shock treatment," or some kind of torture device, but nothing is further from the truth. While ECT is not commonly used, it has proven to be a very structured, very effective way to treat serious cases of antepartum and postpartum depression that do not respond to traditional medication and therapies. Here's how it works: Before ECT, you are given anesthesia to put you in a sleeplike state and medications to relax your muscles. Then an electrical current is briefly sent to the brain through electrodes placed on the temples or elsewhere on the head, depending on the condition being treated and the type of ECT. The electrical stimulation, which lasts up to eight seconds, produces a short, mild seizure. However, the seizure activity related to ECT does not cause the body to convulse. Some people report short-term memory loss, confusion, nausea, headache, and jaw pain immediately following ECT, but these side effects only last a few hours. If you suffer from severe antepartum or postpartum depression and no other treatments have improved your situation, you should seriously consider trying ECT.

Breast-feeding on Medication

If you're breast-feeding, you're probably concerned about how taking antidepressants or antianxiety medications may affect your baby. Until recently, taking medication while nursing wasn't even a question—you simply didn't do it. But in the last five years, several studies have shown that many medications prescribed to treat postpartum depression are reasonably safe to take while breast-feeding your child. That's not to say that there isn't a certain amount of risk involved in exposing your baby to medications—we can't tell you that there's absolutely no risk to your baby's health. But we can tell you that studies show that the risk with certain medications is minimal, and most health professionals agree that treating your PPD and regaining your health and happiness almost always outweigh the potential risks involved with taking medication while nursing. Staying depressed and anxious can have long-term effects on your bond with your baby and your baby's development. Talk with your health-care practitioner about the pros and cons of taking medication while breast-feeding. Together you can decide on the treatment that's right for you.

"I took Zoloft during my pregnancy as well as while I was nursing. I couldn't have done it any other way. I am so grateful for Zoloft. And my son Leo is perfect"

—Judy K.

If you're interested in finding more information on breast-feeding and medication, there are some good books available (see Resources) as well as organizations like Lactation Resource Center Inc. in New Jersey that can assist you with up-to-date information to help you make a decision that you feel comfortable with. Please note that if you decide to stop breast-feeding and begin medication, it's strongly advised that you don't wean too abruptly, as this causes hormonal fluctuations that can affect your emotional well-being (see chapter 3 for more information).

Antidepressants

All antidepressants are excreted in breast milk, but to differing degrees. Multiple case studies suggest that some TCAs and SSRIs can be taken with little risk to your baby. Researchers who've studied the possible impact of Zoloft (sertraline) and Paxil (paroxetine) on breast-fed infants have found no adverse effects. Prozac (fluoxetine) is the only drug "cleared by the FDA" for use during pregnancy, but recent studies have shown that it remains in the bloodstream longer than other antidepressants and may reach higher levels than other antidepressants in breast-fed infants. Prozac has also been linked with irritability, sleep disturbance, and poor feeding in some infants exposed through their mothers' breast milk. Recent studies have also shown that when mothers take Prozac or Paxil during pregnancy and choose not to nurse, their babies may experience withdrawal symptoms, such as respiratory distress, low blood pressure, and jaundice. These studies also show that these babies do not suffer any long-term health effects.

It's important to note that no long-term studies of infants exposed to TCAs and SSRIs through breast milk exist, so health-care practitioners and scientists can't be sure what the long-term effects might be.

Antianxiety Medications

There have been fewer studies done on the relationship between antianxiety medications and breast-feeding, but current research shows that minimal doses of short-acting benzodiazepines such as Klonopin (clonazepam) and Ativan (lorazepam) appear relatively safe. The available data collected on these medications suggest that nursing infants are exposed to low amounts of the drugs through breast milk. Some case reports have been published of sedation, poor feeding, and respiratory distress in nursing infants; however, the data, when pooled, suggest a relatively low incidence of adverse events, particularly when benzodiazepines are used at a low dosage.

If you're currently taking medication while breast-feeding and you feel uncomfortable about it, here's a tip that may help you feel better: Call your health-care practitioner and ask when the medication you're taking peaks in your system. Then use a breast pump to drain your milk at that time and dump it out. This will ensure that your baby is getting the smallest possible amount of medication through your breast milk.

RISK FACTORS OF MEDICATIONS TAKEN WHILE BREAST-FEEDING

LACTATION RISK categories have been assigned to almost all medications by their manufacturers and are based on the level of risk the drug poses to your baby. The FDA has provided these five categories to indicate the risk associated with breast-feeding. As you discuss these drugs with your health-care practitioner, make sure to ask which category they are in.

L1—SAFEST:

Drug that has been taken by a large number of breast-feeding mothers without any observed increase in adverse effects in the infant. Controlled studies in breast-feeding women fail to demonstrate a risk to the infant, and the possibility of harm to the breast-feeding infant is remote or the product is not **orally bioavailable** in an infant.

L2—SAFER:

Drug that has been studied in a limited number of breast-feeding women without an increase in adverse effects in the infant. Or the evidence of a demonstrated risk that is likely to follow use of this medication in a breast-feeding woman is remote.

L3—MODERATELY SAFE:

There are no controlled studies in breast-feeding women; however, the risk of untoward effects to a breast-fed infant is possible, or controlled studies show only minimal nonthreatening adverse effects. Drugs should be given only if the potential benefit justifies the potential risk to the infant.

L4—POSSIBLY HAZARDOUS:

There is positive evidence of risk to a breast-fed infant or to breast milk production, but the benefits from use in breast-feeding mothers may be acceptable despite the risk to the infant (e.g., if the drug is needed in a life-threatening situation or for a serious disease for which safer drugs cannot be used or are ineffective).

L5—CONTRAINDICATED:

Studies in breast-feeding mothers have demonstrated that there is significant and documented risk to the infant based on human experience, or it is a medication that has a high risk of causing significant damage to an infant. The risk of using the drug in breast-feeding women clearly outweighs any possible benefit from breast-feeding. The drug is contraindicated in women who are breast-feeding an infant.

The Therapies

Though it's sometimes possible to treat your postpartum depression without medication, therapy is *always* crucial to your recovery. This means your recovery will most likely be something of a team effort, involving at least two medical professionals who will help you through the process and monitor your progress. The fact is, a combination of medication and psychotherapy will usually help you work through your postpartum depression faster and more completely than a single type of treatment, which will lower your chances of developing PPD again with subsequent pregnancies.

Finding the Right Therapist

There are several types of health-care professionals who are qualified to provide therapy for postpartum depression:

Psychologist. Psychologists are health professionals with training and expertise in human behavior and psychological health. They are not medical doctors, but they hold a doctor of psychology (PsyD) or doctor of philosophy (PhD) in clinical psychology, counseling, or school psychology.

Psychologists evaluate and treat people who have mental health problems, such as depression. Psychologists also provide counseling and other mental health services. In most states, psychologists do not prescribe medication. However, many states are reviewing prescription-writing privileges for psychologists, and regulations may change. Some psychologists practicing in New Mexico, Louisiana, the territory of Guam, the U.S. military, Indian Health Services, and other departments of the federal government have prescription privileges.

Social worker. Social workers are health professionals who use counseling to help people function in their environment, improve their relationships with others, and solve personal and family problems. They also help people locate and access appropriate resources for their particular needs.

A social worker may work in a hospital, community organization, or private counseling, and most of them concentrate on a specific area of practice.

Advanced practice nurse. An advanced practice nurse is first educated as a registered professional nurse then continues with additional graduate education in psychiatric mental health nursing at the masters or doctoral level. Usually the American Nurses' Association nationally certifies him or her in Psychiatric–Mental Health Nursing. This requires passing a national examination and remaining current through continuing education and recertification procedures. In many states, advanced practice nurses can prescribe medications.

Licensed professional counselor. Mental health counselors provide counseling services for individuals, couples, families, teens, and children. Mental health counselors must earn a master's degree in counseling or a closely related mental health field and complete a minimum of two years of clinical work after earning their degree. Many licensed mental health counselors are also social workers or psychologists who hold a doctoral degree.

Psychiatrist. As mentioned in the "Finding the Right Health Professional" section in chapter 3, psychiatrists are medical doctors who specialize in the diagnosis and treatment of mental health problems. They can prescribe medications to treat mental illness, and some provide counseling.

What to Look for in a Therapist

Because therapy is such an intimate process, it's essential that you feel comfortable with your therapist so that you can develop an open and trusting relationship that will facilitate growth and progress. The health professional who diagnosed you with PPD may be able to provide you with the names of some therapists who have experience treating postpartum depression. If not, you can visit the Postpartum Support International Web site (www.postpartum.net) and click on the "PSI Coordinators" link on the home page. There you'll find the contact information for the PSI coordinator for your state, who can put you in touch with therapists who specialize in postpartum depression treatment in your area. See the box on page 108 for more tips on finding a therapist in your area.

Once you've gotten the contact information for a therapist you'd like to try, we suggest you briefly interview her by phone or face-to-face. Ask questions. Listen to your feelings and trust your intuition. Don't hesitate to change your mind and seek another provider if you don't feel satisfied. It's important to select someone who fits your personality style.

Here are some questions to ask during your interview:

- What type of license do you have?
- What are your credentials or certifications?
- Tell me about your experience with mothers who have had postpartum mood disorders.
- How do you feel about women with PPD?
- How many women with PPD have you treated?
- Are you up-to-date on current information about PPD?
- What type of therapy do you practice?
- What are your scheduled office hours, and how available are you?
- Do you offer any support groups?
- Will you provide me with information I can take home to read?
- If you are away, do you have someone who can take your place?
- Can I contact you twenty-four hours a day in case of an emergency?
- How long are your sessions?
- Can I bring my baby or other children to sessions?

Be sure to discuss fees, insurance, and emergency care up front, before you begin treatment. You should also call your insurance company and find out exactly what they'll cover with regard to therapy. Mental health coverage varies, and you may find that your insurance company will authorize only a limited number of sessions. This is important because it's possible that completing your treatment may mean having to go beyond the number of sessions that your health insurance is willing to permit. To remedy this situation, there is a process of appeal with some insurance companies that you may be able to utilize. But remember this: your mental health is one of the most important investments you can make in the future of you and your child, so it's worth every penny. A lot of therapists are flexible when it comes to payment for services, so don't be afraid to talk to yours about the possibility of a sliding scale, payment plan, or other alternative ways to make payments.

HOW TO FIND A THERAPIST IN YOUR AREA

THERE IS one national organization that provides names of therapists in your area who specialize in postpartum depression:

Postpartum Support International
www.postpartum.net

Keep in mind that Postpartum Support International is not endorsing the therapists on its list. They're simply offering you the names of professionals who have identified themselves as specialists in PPD.
Here are some other ideas:

- Ask your obstetrician or your baby's pediatrician for recommendations.
- If you have any friends or family members who have seen a therapist, ask for the therapist's contact information and give her a call. She may not have any experience with postpartum depression, but she may know someone who does and can refer you.
- the group coordinator of your local PPD support group (if there is one) and ask her to recommend a therapist in your area.
- If there's a new mother support group in your area, call the group coordinator and ask if she has a list of mental-health professionals she can share.
- Some states provide state-run programs for PPD. Call your state's

Health and Human Services Department and ask for some recommendations.

- Find out if your state has a Self-Help Clearinghouse, which is a statewide organization that provides information on all support groups in your state. If so, call their toll-free number and get the contact information for the PPD support groups nearest you. Then call the support group leaders and ask for recommendations.
- Check your local newspaper or YMCA or community center bulletin for postings about support groups.

Types of Therapy

There are several different types of therapy that can be beneficial to you as you work through your postpartum depression. There are no "cookie-cutter" PPD patients, and the best approach to recovery is one that is designed to suit your individual needs. Your therapy will be multifaceted and may include elements of more than one of the therapies we describe below.

Talk Therapy

Talk therapy is exactly what it sounds like—talking with a therapist about what is bothering you. Talking about your problems can help you to spot issues that are causing problems in your life. A person with a different perspective on your situation can help you decide how to fix the problems you are having, and how to deal with those you can't fix. Through discussion, you can find ways to handle your problems so that the same issues won't continually disrupt your life.

There are three common types of talk therapy used in treating postpartum depression: cognitive therapy, behavioral therapy, and interpersonal therapy.

COGNITIVE THERAPY

Cognitive therapy helps you change harmful ways of thinking. If you tend to see things negatively, it teaches you how to look at the world more clearly. Cognitive therapy can be conducted in a group setting or on an individual basis. Typically, cognitive therapy is very structured and lasts approximately ten to fifteen weeks. This is important to note, because women with postpartum depression almost always need longer than the ten to fifteen weeks of treatment.

In order to benefit from cognitive therapy, you need to be motivated and willing to do weekly assignments, such as recording situations, moods, and automatic thoughts along with the dates they occurred. For example, perhaps one day you go to the mall and your baby starts crying uncontrollably. You would detail the situation in a journal and describe your mood at the time, how you felt, and what you were thinking. For the sake of this example we'll say you felt like a failure. Then you would come up with evidence to support an alternative thought, or why you are not a failure. Perhaps the baby was crying because she had gas, you were able to calm her down after a little while, you did the best you could, and so forth. The goal of cognitive therapy is to help you see that you are learning to be a good mother.

BEHAVIORAL THERAPY

Behavioral therapy helps you change harmful ways of acting. The goal is to gain control over behavior that is causing problems for you. Behavioral therapy helps you trace the problematic thought and change it. Say, for example, that you have it in your head that the light switch must be on at all times in the bathroom. Where did this belief come from? Perhaps when you were growing up your mother used to tell you that the light had to stay on. Now you reexamine that belief. Does it really have to be on? You might try one night to leave it off and see what happens. You then realize that it's fine to turn off the light, and you begin to change this learned behavior.

INTERPERSONAL THERAPY

Interpersonal therapy helps you learn to relate better to others. You'll focus on how to express your feelings and how to develop better people skills. Like cognitive behavioral therapy, interpersonal therapy is often short term, but it can also be ongoing. It focuses on practical issues. The American Psychiatric Association says that the benefits of interpersonal therapy are well established by many studies.

In fact, one small 2001 study published in the *American Journal of Psychiatry* showed that among women who were involved in interpersonal therapy during their pregnancies, the risk of postpartum depression was significantly reduced.

Therapy isn't just useful for people who are working through emotional problems, and you don't have to stop going to therapy when your postpartum depression is resolved. Lots of people stay in therapy for the extra support it provides and as a preemptive measure, so that they don't get sick. Going to therapy is an educated choice that people make to improve their lives, mature more quickly, and cope with life more effectively.

Group Therapy

Group therapy is another type of psychotherapy that can be useful for postpartum depression. Led by a professional, group therapy is a way of getting help along with other people who are recovering from the same condition. Unlike the talk therapies we described above, group therapy is never used for deep-seated conflict resolution. You are generally required to have been in individual therapy for at least a year before starting group therapy so that you are no longer in "crisis" and so that everyone in the group is in roughly the same stage of recovery. Group therapy is also less costly than individual therapy.

There are many benefits to group therapy. First, it can help you realize that you're not alone in how you're feeling or what you're thinking. All the other women participating in the group are going through a similar experience, and it can be a great relief to hear others talk about thoughts and feelings that you may be afraid to verbalize. Group therapy helps foster realistic beliefs and encourages socialization. It helps women become more aware of and gain insight into their behavioral patterns so that they can change behaviors that don't work.

Group therapy is also a very comfortable and safe atmosphere that doesn't force self-disclosure. The women support one another through the process, trading tips and offering suggestions to help one another cope and improve their situations. The encouragement you receive to keep moving forward in group therapy can be invaluable as you work to get your life back on track.

What to Expect from Your Therapist

In order to get a full picture of what you're going through and to get to know you better, your therapist will ask you a lot of questions. Initial visits typically take up to two hours, which is about the time it will take for your therapist to do a full initial evaluation. You'll be asked about your symptoms and when they started. You'll be asked about your family history and whether you've ever been diagnosed with any mood disorders or other psychiatric conditions. You'll also need to be prepared to talk about your marriage, your family, and the stressors in your life. Your therapist will likely want to discuss your sleeping patterns, your eating habits, your experiences during pregnancy, labor, and delivery, and more—anything that might have some bearing on PPD. Some of these questions may be uncomfortable or embarrassing for you, but this is a necessary step in your recovery, so be open and honest with your therapist.

The primary focus of your therapy should be on relieving your current postpartum depression symptoms. This is not the time to solve historical and long-standing issues, such as conflict in your family. Your therapist's job is to help you work through your PPD and develop healthy lifestyle changes and coping mechanisms. The time for delving into your past (if you wish to pursue it) is after your PPD has been resolved. As Joyce likes to say, your therapist needs to put out the fire first (your postpartum depression) and then sift through the ashes to see how your past may have added to the fire. Examining the past while a patient is still symptomatic usually only adds to her agitation and other symptoms. That said, we do encourage you to address any issues from your past when the time is right in order to reduce your future risk for PPD or other emotional problems.

The goal of your therapy is for you to become yourself again but to be better at being yourself than ever before. A good therapist looks at her patients holistically—therapy should be a total mind and body experience, with no stone left unturned.

It's also important to remember that therapy is a service that you are paying for, so you need to get your money's worth. Therapy has to work for you, and you must feel comfortable with your therapist. Don't be afraid to try a new therapist if you have any reservations about the person you are seeing now.

How Long Should Therapy Last?

Every woman's condition is different, so there is no set length of time that you should be in therapy for PPD. Therapy for postpartum depression typically lasts a year, but it should always last as long as you and your therapist think is necessary. There are also other factors that affect the length of therapy. For instance, some women have other emotional issues in addition to postpartum depression, and they may very well need to stay in therapy longer than a year. Many women who have healed from their PPD choose to continue therapy as a preemptive measure. Others continue to go to therapy a few times a year for a "tune-up," or as a safe place to go for a reality check.

Alternative Therapies

Many Americans, especially women, use alternative medicine to treat all types of ailments. One of the main reasons why women with post-partum depression may seek alternative medicine treatments is that they are concerned about the effects of pharmacological treatment on breast-feeding. Many alternative treatments are inexpensive, accessible, and generally safe and well tolerated, which makes them attractive options for treating PPD. Anecdotal evidence does show that women suffering from postpartum depression may benefit from several inter-ventions other than medications and psychotherapy. However, it's important to note that although research has been done on the use of alternative medicine in treating depression, and more studies are in progress, almost no studies have addressed their use in postpartum depression in particular.

Below we've described the alternative treatments that some women have found beneficial. Keep in mind that all of these treatments should be used in conjunction with traditional medical treatment as ways to help relieve and cope with your symptoms. None of these practices alone will end your postpartum depression. If you decide to try an alternative form of therapy, be sure to inform your health-care providers so that they can adjust their treatments if necessary.

Acupuncture

Acupuncture balances the flow of chi, or energy, and blood through-out your body, which can help resolve the underlying energetic imbalance that is contributing to your postpartum depression. Stimulating acupuncture points has been shown to release endorphins and **enkephalins**. Hence, acupuncture treatments can have a calming, mood-elevating effect. If you are suffering physical symptoms in conjunction with your PPD, such as headache, stomachache, or back-ache, acupuncture can help to alleviate them. You should consult a professional acupuncturist for this treatment.

Biofeedback

Anecdotal evidence suggests that biofeedback is effective in reducing the intensity of all types of depression. It attempts to change brain wave patterns through training, essentially doing what drugs do chemically.

Biofeedback training is a systematized approach for learning relax-ation that furnishes feedback evidence of reaching a calmer level of brain wave activity and physiological response. By allowing you to focus your energy in a self-empowering way, it gives you a greater feeling of control over your autonomic nervous system reactions (heart rate, blood pressure), including those triggered by stress. You get hooked up to apparatus that measures your responses (heart rate, muscle tension, skin temperature, brain waves) while you focus on a sensory cue to help you relax. Learning to relax on cue can be a huge help when dealing with the anxiety that often accompanies PPD.

Exercise

Exercise is essential for both physical and mental health. It provides an outlet for releasing negative emotions, such as anger, frustration, and irritability. By stimulating the production of neurotransmitters in the brain, such as norepinephrine, exercise can help to lift you out of a depressive funk.

Physical activity should be a part of any therapy for depression. Even if used alone, exercise can often bring startling results. Studies show that jogging for thirty minutes three times a week can be as effective as psychotherapy in treating depression. Any exercise is fine; the more energetic and aerobic, the better.

Light Therapy

Light therapy is exposure to light that is brighter than indoor light but not as bright as direct sunlight. It is most commonly used to treat seasonal affective disorder (SAD), which is depression related to shorter days and reduced sunlight exposure during the fall and winter months, but some women have also found it to be helpful during their postpartum depression.

A good way to enjoy the benefits of light therapy without spending a lot of money is to buy natural lightbulbs and install them around your home. Many hardware stores sell them and they're quite inexpensive. You can also purchase them online at www.bulbs.com.

Massage Therapy

Massage uses touch to provide relaxation. While there are variations of massage, they all work under the general principle of the connection between body and mind—that when the body is relaxed and at ease, the mind is promoting better health, less depression, and overall well-being. If you're pregnant, be sure to get the OK from your health-care practitioner before getting a massage, and tell the massage therapist you are pregnant. There are pressure points on your wrists and ankles that can stimulate the uterus and possibly induce contractions, so your massage therapist needs to know he must avoid them. Ideally you should make an appointment with someone who has been trained to give prenatal massages. She will know exactly how to make you feel good and will be set up with the right equipment (massage table specially made for pregnant women, pillows, etc.) to meet your needs.

Meditation

Meditation has a very calming affect. It helps to ease tension and improves your capacity to concentrate. As you meditate, you also become much more attuned to your inner feelings and sensations, achieving a heightened state of awareness. Rather than dwelling on the negative emotions that are making you feel depressed, you can transcend them through meditation. This kind of personal growth, in which you gain a higher level of consciousness and greater awareness of yourself, can help to bolster your self-confidence, self-esteem, and peace of mind. Your mind is free to travel beyond the busy chatter of thoughts to a silent, tranquil place. In turn, a positive emotional outlook and sense of well-being can help you maintain good physical and mental health.

Spirituality

A recent survey done by the National Center for Alternative and Complementary Medicine found that prayer was by far the most commonly used method among complementary and alternative therapies. It's difficult to pinpoint what prayer can do for the ailing, but studies show that people who attend religious services or pray regularly are happier people and are better able to cope with stress and disease. Your spiritual beliefs and feelings should also be an important part of your treatment plan.

Reflexology

This is a technique in which a therapist applies pressure to specific points on the hands and feet. Reflexologists believe that the body has the capacity to heal itself. There are nerves in the hands and feet that are related to various parts of the body, and by manipulating these points through reflexology it is thought that the healing process is stimulated. Pregnant women should stay away from reflexology, as many of the pressure points used can stimulate the uterus and possibly induce contractions.

Yoga

Yoga is a relaxing form of exercise that tones the nervous system, stimulates circulation, promotes concentration, and energizes your mind and body. Yoga stretching exercises also help improve blood circulation, making it easier to break through the lethargy that often accompanies depression.

Retail Therapy

Go shopping. Treat yourself to something nice (but affordable). We swear by it—it never fails to make us feel better.

SIX

Taking Care
of Yourself

IN ADDITION TO taking medication and talking with a therapist, taking good care of yourself will make your recovery from postpartum depression quicker and easier. Many women feel they don't have the time or energy to nurture themselves after they've met the demands of the baby, other children, a job, and the household chores. Others think it's wrong to put their needs before the needs of their loved ones. But taking care of your own needs when you have postpartum depression is crucial to your recovery, not an option or a luxury. There is a direct link between what you do, how you sleep, eat, and exercise, and how you feel emotionally. Thinking of self-care as a requirement for getting better can help ease any guilt you may feel about taking the time to do it.

Educate Yourself

We are firm believers in the importance of being proactive about your health. Now that you know you're suffering from postpartum depression, you should learn everything you can about the condition. Arming yourself with knowledge will make you better prepared to work with your health-care practitioners to come up with the best treatment for you. Knowing the nature of your illness will make you better able to work through it and put it behind you. You've gotten off to a good start by picking up this book, but don't stop there.

1. Search the Internet for articles, studies, and reputable Web sites dedicated to the topic. You can also find thousands of personal stories from women who want to share their experiences on the Internet. These stories are often moving, always interesting, and will give you a real glimpse into how other women have dealt with (and are dealing with) PPD.

2. Go to your local library and see what they have available on the topic of postpartum depression or perinatal mood disorders. Also check the library's community calendar and their local resource guide for PPD support groups.

3. If you know someone who has been through postpartum depression, take a chance and talk to her about it. Ask questions. Regardless of whether or not they've gone "public," women who've had PPD are often more than happy to discuss it when they know they're helping someone deal with what they've been through themselves.

Also see the Resources section on page 218 for books and Web sites you may find interesting.

Get Plenty of Rest

You need your rest to fight fatigue and depression, but the months after having a baby will probably be the *least* restful of your life. Although you probably won't get eight consecutive hours for a while, we strongly suggest that you strive for a minimum of four hours of "good," uninterrupted sleep. In addition, here are some suggestions you can try to ensure you're getting as much rest as you can.

1. **Sleep whenever your baby does.** We're sure you've heard this one before, but napping with your baby really is the best way to catch up on your sleep and preserve your strength. Your baby will probably eat every two to three hours for the first few months of his life, which means you will be seriously sleep deprived unless you figure out another way to get some sleep. Taking advantage of the times when your baby sleeps by sleeping at those times yourself will help you feel stronger, more alert, more in control, and more optimistic during the tough times. If you have difficulty sleeping because of anxiety, depression, or racing thoughts, talk to your health-care practitioner.

2. **If you can't sleep, then use the time to relax.** Some women find it difficult to fall asleep while their baby is napping. If that's the case for you, then at least use this time to relax. Lie down on your bed and close your eyes for a while. Or get comfortable on your sofa and watch some mindless TV, nothing upsetting or disturbing. Just make sure that whatever you're doing is not work. It's very tempting to use the time when your baby is napping to catch up on housework, make phone calls, or write those overdue thank-you notes, but all of that can wait. There is nothing more important than getting as much rest as you can in the first months after your baby is born. When your baby gets a little older, starts sleeping longer, and you're feeling stronger, then you can begin to try phasing in some work while he naps. But until then, let the dishes and the laundry pile up. You can't accomplish everything you could before your baby arrived—it's physically impossible, so don't even try. Give yourself a break and let your partner pick up the slack for a while.

3. **Take breaks throughout the day.** People take breaks all the time in the working world in order to relieve stress and relax a little, which makes them more productive at their jobs. The law actually requires breaks for workers. Well, mothering is no different. Every few hours, sit down and unwind for a few minutes. Put your feet up and enjoy a glass of cold iced tea. Read a magazine or a few pages from a book you've been chipping

away at. Or just close your eyes, take some deep breaths, and try to clear your mind.

Seek Support at Home

Taking care of the baby, doing the housework and the laundry, cooking meals, running errands—there's a lot to do to keep your household running smoothly, and you just can't do it all by yourself right now. You're going through a huge adjustment and tending to a baby who needs almost constant attention. Trying to accomplish everything you used to be able to handle will cause you a lot of unnecessary stress and frustration and will worsen your PPD symptoms. Ask your family and friends to give you a hand until you get back on your feet again. Here are some suggestions for how they can help you:

- Ask your partner to give the baby one or two of his nighttime feedings. Even if you're breast-feeding, you can pump some milk during the day and have your partner bottle-feed your baby during the night. This will give you a chance to sleep more than just an hour or two at a time, or to just relax while someone else does a feeding for you.
- Have a friend or a family member come with you when you have to run errands. She can watch the baby while you do what you need to do more quickly and with less stress.
- Have a friend or family member come over to watch the baby when you don't have errands to run so that you can catch up on sleep.
- Ask your mom to help you with the laundry once a week. If you're feeling energetic, maybe you can put the clothes in the washer and dryer and then your mom can fold them for you.
- Ask your partner to help with the dishes when they start to pile up. If you don't have a dishwasher, perhaps he can wash and you could dry.
- If you have an older child, put her to work. Ask her to put the toys away in the living room, or to straighten up her room. You could even make a game of it—if she picks up all

her toys in less than five minutes she can pick out a book for you to read to her when the baby is napping (or anything that you know will make her happy).

Another way to get the help you need during this transitional time is to hire a housekeeper. Not everyone can afford to do this, but since it would only be for a few months, it's a viable option for some. A housekeeper could keep your house clean, do your laundry for you, and even cook some of your meals. This way you can focus your energy on taking care of your baby and regaining your strength. It would make it a lot easier to find time for yourself and time for rest as well (see chapter 7 for more ideas and information).

HOW DO YOU SPEND YOUR TIME?

IF YOU'RE feeling guilty or ashamed about needing help, here's a good way to put your needs in perspective. Use the circle below to create a pie chart depicting your answers to the following questions.

What percentage of your day do you spend:

1. doing for others in your family?
2. doing for others outside your family?
3. doing for yourself?
4. having significant others do for you?

You've probably found that you spend almost all of your time doing for others. Let your friends and family return the favor.

Develop a Social Support Network

Getting together with other mothers who share similar concerns and needs has been shown to help ease the effects of postpartum depression. Once you realize that you are not alone in your struggles, that other women are going through the same feelings and experiences as you are, it will drive home the fact that there is absolutely nothing wrong with you. So one of the best things you can do for yourself is to make friends with other parents. Here are some ways to do that:

- Join a Mommy and Me class at your local community center or YMCA.
- Sign up for story time at your town library.
- Join a Mothers of Multiples group.
- Try Gymboree.
- Sign up for a Music Together class.
- Join a Moms Club.
- Join the postpartum support group provided by your hospital.
- Join playgroups with other new mothers, or form your own group.
- Even if your baby is too young to appreciate it, take him to the playground and strike up conversations with other moms.

If you already have friends with children, reach out and give them a call. Ask them about their experiences. Ask them for advice on how to handle some of the issues you've been struggling with. Talk about how you're feeling. This is a great way to get some perspective on your situation, to learn new ways of doing things, and discover resources for you and your child. Other moms usually have a wealth of knowledge about classes you can take, good babysitters, and shortcuts that will make life easier. You can also ask them to babysit for you while you get some much-needed rest or have an hour of "me" time. You'll be much more comfortable having someone you know and trust watch over your baby, and other mothers know better than anyone how important it is to have some time off.

Make Time for Yourself

It's really difficult to go from being responsible for only yourself to caring for an infant. You don't realize how important your free time was until it's gone. Remember when you could lie down for a few minutes whenever you wanted to, or spend the whole day shopping, or just laze around on a rainy Sunday? All of those things helped you de-stress and recharge, and you need those types of outlets now more than ever. It's imperative that you find a way to make time for yourself. You may no longer be able to spend a lazy Sunday on the couch watching TV, but there are plenty of activities you can do that take less time and will make you happy. Anything you enjoy will do the trick—read, go for a walk, take a bath, do something creative. Just make sure you're doing it alone. Spending some time away from your baby is *good* for you, so try not to feel guilty about it.

Leave the House

Staying home all day long, every day, is not good for you. Contact with others and changes of scenery will help you feel more connected to the world and elevate your mood. It's a good idea to make a plan for each day, either the night before or in the morning when you wake up, that will get you out of the house for a while. Take your baby for a walk around the neighborhood. Go into town and get a coffee (decaffeinated, of course!). Drive to your parents' house for a visit. Meet your friend and her dog at the park. Just get out of the house every day, even if it's just for fifteen minutes—isolation often perpetuates depression.

Exercise

Getting into an exercise routine after the birth of your baby is beneficial for several reasons. First and foremost, exercise is a proven way to elevate your mood when you're feeling depressed or anxious. As you already know, serotonin is an important neurotransmitter in the brain that has been linked to depression. Some researchers have found that regular exercise, and the resulting increase in physical fitness, alters serotonin levels and leads to improved mood and feelings of well-being. Research also indicates that regular exercise boosts body temperature, which may ease depression by influencing serotonin and other neurotransmitters.

Regular exercise has obvious physical benefits as well. It can take several months for your body to snap back after pregnancy, and many women feel extremely unhappy and stressed about their post-pregnancy body. Feeling overweight, out of shape, or unattractive and being unable to fit into your pre-pregnancy clothes can take a toll on your confidence, which will only contribute to your postpartum depression. Exercise will help you shed that lingering baby weight and return your body to its normal size and condition a lot faster. You'll also be improving your cardiovascular health, reducing your cholesterol level and blood pressure, and generally extending your life.

Exercise will also help you boost your self-esteem. Physical activity makes you feel good about yourself. You're taking an active role in getting into shape and improving your health. If you participate in group sports, the social aspect of getting together with a group of people on a regular basis can be a great confidence booster. An important note: be sure to clear it with your health-care practitioner before you start an exercise regimen, even if you exercised through your pregnancy. Women who've had C-sections typically must wait six to eight weeks before they can become physically active again. You should also start out slowly, exercising maybe fifteen minutes at a time for the first few weeks, and work your way up to thirty or forty-five minutes of activity. The last thing you want to do is injure yourself.

Choosing the best cardiovascular exercise is easy—if you just do what you enjoy, you'll be more motivated to exercise consistently. Try to keep things fresh and interesting by changing your routine often or doing more than one type of cardio in a session. For example, if you work out at a gym, you could spend fifteen minutes on the treadmill, fifteen minutes on the stationary bicycle, and fifteen minutes on the elliptical machine instead of spending the entire forty-five minutes on the treadmill. If you still have trouble getting yourself to exercise, ask a friend to work out with you. It'll be harder to miss that workout session, and having a workout buddy makes exercise more fun. We know you're crunched for time, so here's a list of the top ten cardio exercises that will get you into great shape and burn the most calories in thirty minutes:

1. **Step Aerobics.** Step aerobics mainly target your legs, hips, and glutes and can burn approximately 400 calories in 30 minutes.
2. **Bicycling.** Both stationary and outdoor bicycling are great cardio exercises. Depending on the resistance and speed, you can burn 250 to 500 calories in 30 minutes.
3. **Swimming.** Swimming is an excellent full-body exercise. Doing the breaststroke can burn approximately 400 calories in 30 minutes.
4. **Racquetball.** Side-to-side sprinting makes racquetball an excellent cardio exercise. A 145-pound person burns over 400 calories in 30 minutes.
5. **Rock Climbing.** Rock climbing isn't just a cardio exercise; it also uses arm and leg strength and power. You can burn up to 380 calories in 30 minutes.
6. **Cross-Country Skiing.** Whether on a machine or outdoors on snow, cross-country skiing is an incredible cardio exercise, because it requires you to use both your upper and lower body. A 145-pound person can burn approximately 330 calories in 30 minutes.
7. **Running.** Running is a great cardio workout, because all you need is a pair of quality running shoes. Running burns serious calories. A 145-pound person can easily burn 300 calories in 30 minutes.
8. **Elliptical Trainer.** The elliptical provides low-impact cardio exercise that also offers a great way to build endurance. A 145-pound person can burn about 300 calories in 30 minutes.
9. **Rowing.** Rowing gives your arms an incredible workout. A 145-pound person can burn about 300 calories in 30 minutes.
10. **Walking.** Brisk walking is a less strenuous form of cardio. Walking can burn up to 180 calories in 30 minutes. Sprinting or adding hills or an incline will increase the amount of calories burned.

Of course, it may be hard or even impossible for you to have someone watch your baby while you exercise. Here are some exercise ideas you can do with your baby:

1. Put your baby in a stroller and take her for a walk around your neighborhood or into town.
2. Buy a jogging stroller and take your baby along with you on your runs. Jogging strollers can be expensive (anywhere from $150 to $350), but buying one is a good investment if you use it a couple of times a week. If the price tag sounds too steep, you could also buy a used jogging stroller from a consignment shop that carries baby gear or even online from sites like Ebay.
3. Go to your local YMCA or fitness center and look into group classes for mothers and babies. Most of them offer a pretty good variety, from swim classes to gymnastics to yoga.
4. If you're interested in yoga or Pilates, look in the Yellow Pages or do an online search for studios in your area that are solely dedicated to one of these disciplines. They will often offer postnatal classes where you can bring your baby along.
5. If you are so inclined, sex is considered exercise.

Here are some ideas for team activities in which you could participate:

1. Call your local YMCA or community center and ask if they sponsor team activities like soccer or tennis.
2. Many companies put together softball teams in the spring and summer months and play against other local companies. If your company does this, consider getting involved.
3. Many bars and local stores sponsor softball teams as well. Visit your favorite watering hole or store and ask if they have a team.
4. Many YMCAs offer a Masters swimming program that you can join for usually a nominal fee. Masters swimming teams typically practice a few times a week and compete against other Masters teams in the area.
5. Churches and other houses of worship often sponsor softball,

dodgeball, basketball, volleyball, soccer, and other sports leagues that you could join.

These are just a few of the many ways you can incorporate exercise into your life—there are dozens of other activities you could do that qualify as a workout, such as hiking or in-line skating. Any type of physical exercise will do. The important thing is that you get moving.

Eat Nutritiously

Your diet plays a significant role in how you feel. Poor nutrition is common among women with postpartum depression, and it is now more important than ever for you to maintain good physical health. Women with PPD usually either overindulge in high carbohydrate and high sugar foods in an unconscious attempt to self medicate, or they have no appetite at all and experience rapid weight loss. Both of these patterns can make your postpartum depression symptoms worse. Insufficient nutrition can cause fatigue, and eating "bad foods" can lower your self-esteem, because you know you shouldn't be eating them but you do it anyway. We recommend that you eat either six small meals or three meals and three snacks a day to maintain your blood sugar level. Here are some tips for eating as nutritiously as possible:

Eat a variety of whole grains. Complex carbohydrates are good for you and will help you feel full for longer. When you have a sandwich, make it on whole-grain bread. For breakfast, substitute Cheerios, Total, or oatmeal in place of sugary cereals. Eat brown rice or wild rice instead of white rice. Popcorn is a good whole-grain snack. Just make sure you buy the lightly buttered kind.

Eat plenty of fruits and vegetables. Have your partner cut up some veggies that you can grab when you get the urge to snack. Or buy the precut veggies at your grocery store. Baby carrots are great to munch on. Most grocery stores also carry premade salads—all you need to do is rinse it, dump it in a bowl, and you have a nutritious lunch or accompaniment to dinner.

Fruits are easy—just make sure you have them on hand and that they're easily accessible. Keep bananas and apples in a bowl on your counter and grapes front and center in your refrigerator.

Choose lean meats and fish. When you're shopping for meat, buy the leanest cuts you can. It's fine to have that hamburger, but make sure it's no more than 15 percent fat. Choose skinless chicken and turkey. Beef and pork tenderloin and lamb chops are also good lean meat choices.

Fish that are high in **omega-3 fatty acids** are great for you. Have at least two servings of baked or grilled fish each week, especially oily fish like salmon or tuna. (Some types of fish may contain high levels of mercury, PCBs [polychlorinated biphenyls,] dioxins, and other environmental contaminants. If you're nursing, avoid shark, swordfish, tilefish [golden bass or golden snapper], and king mackerel.)

Stay away from caffeine, alcohol, sugar, and salt. Large amounts of sugar can cause mood changes that are severe enough to affect your work and concentration. It also causes rapid swings in your blood sugar levels that can trigger panic attacks. Caffeine can trigger both anxiety and mood changes, and can contribute to insomnia, so you should avoid it. Salt can cause fluid retention and electrolyte imbalance, which can affect your mood. Alcohol and other drugs can also affect your mood adversely. You don't have to abstain from alcohol altogether—an occasional drink is fine—but it's best to have no more than one or two drinks a week.

If you have no appetite, here are some ideas for stimulating your appetite and getting the calories and nutrients you need:

Try comfort foods. You may have some luck with the comfort foods that have made you feel better in the past. Grilled cheese sandwiches, macaroni and cheese, chicken noodle soup, pizza, milkshakes, and ice cream are all good choices. Joyce keeps a supply of Hershey's Kisses in her office for her patients.

Limit drinks during meals. Liquids can fill you up and limit your intake of higher calorie foods. It may help to drink most of your liquids thirty to sixty minutes before or after meals.

Try nutritional supplement drinks. Boost or Boost Plus, Carnation Instant Breakfast, and Ensure or Ensure Plus, among other nutritional beverages, can provide a significant amount of calories and require little or no preparation. It may be easier for you to drink rather than to eat your calories.

Experiment with different foods. Once-favorite foods may no longer appeal to you, while foods you were never fond of may become more appealing. So try a bite of something you may not normally choose.

Spend Time Alone with Your Partner

You need to nurture your connection with your partner, especially now, when you need his support the most. Make an effort to spend time alone together. If you feel comfortable leaving your baby with a sitter, go out and have a nice, quiet dinner together. Or you could stay home, order takeout, and eat together while your baby is sleeping. It doesn't matter what you do as long as you're doing it together. The important thing is to talk with your partner about how you are feeling. He needs to understand what's going on with you in order to help you through this, and just talking with someone you trust can provide some relief. Spending time alone with your partner does not necessarily mean you have to have sex. You can be intimate without sex, using hand-holding, massage, or taking quiet walks together. This will help you feel better about your relationship and more connected to each other (see chapter 9 for a detailed discussion about sex).

Keep a Journal

Writing down your feelings and emotions is a great way to release them. You don't need to be a writer or even to have kept a journal before to start one now. Just buy a lined notebook at the grocery store or pharmacy. Or if you think it will encourage you to write consistently, you could go to the bookstore and buy a bound journal with a lovely cover. You can be as descriptive or as simple as you want to be, but make sure you dedicate at least a few minutes each day to writing in it. Here are some ideas on what to write about:

- How you felt that day—was it a good day or a bad one? Did you feel sad, overwhelmed, angry, hopeful, or happy? If you think you know what prompted you to feel certain things, include that as well.
- What went well during the day, and how did it make you feel? Hopeful? Strong? In control?
- What frustrated or angered you during the day?
- How is your baby doing generally? How is she eating and sleeping?
- What did you accomplish during the day? (Remember, even showers are an accomplishment!)

You could also keep a gratitude journal, in which you write down what you are grateful for each day. Journals can be especially useful as you recover, because you can reread them to see how far you've come.

Have Realistic Expectations of Yourself and Others

It's common and normal for new moms to have unrealistic expectations of themselves, their babies, their partners, their family, their friends, and their lives, particularly new moms with postpartum depression. Women with PPD are typically high achievers and perfectionists who believe that they can handle everything themselves and "do it all," which is an impossible feat to expect of yourself after having a baby. It can be difficult to change this type of negative thinking and behavior into positive thoughts and behaviors, but holding on to your unrealistic expectations will make it much more difficult for you to adjust during your postpartum period.

First of all, don't be too hard on yourself. Mothering is a learned skill, and you will make mistakes, just as every other mother on the planet has. Try to be as relaxed as you can when things go wrong or not as you expected. You should also be careful not to pressure yourself to do as much as you did before your baby was born. Your life is ruled by your baby now, and it is simply impossible for you to function at the same level as you did before the baby arrived. Life is a lot harder now. Scale back your expectations for the perfect household. Do what you can and leave the rest. Ask for help when you need it. You don't have to keep up appearances; set a goal to get one task done each day—this is a step in the right direction—and remember, there may be days when you can't get anything done, and that's perfectly normal and fine.

Many women daydream about how their babies will look and act when they're born, and the reality is often very different. This can lead to feelings of disappointment and guilt. Try to accept your baby as she is. Remind yourself that your baby's looks and behavior will change a great deal over the next several months. Express your feelings to your therapist so that she can help you realize that these feelings are normal.

Many women are resentful of their partners because they feel that the baby has changed their lives drastically but that their partners' lives haven't changed at all. This isn't exactly true—your partner is going through an adjustment period as well, just not as radical as yours. If this is your first baby, then your partner really is experiencing many of the same feelings as you are. Do your best to keep the lines of communication open. Be clear and honest about your needs and concerns. Don't expect him to know what you are thinking or what you need if you haven't told him.

Your friends are certainly there to help you, but they have their own lives to lead as well. You should absolutely ask them to give you a hand when you need it, but don't expect that they'll always be able to do what you want. Understand that this doesn't make them any less your friend. Remember, they have their own commitments to take care of, their own children to deal with, and their own problems to solve.

Sometimes having a baby can change the dynamic of your friendship with someone, especially if your friend doesn't have children. It can be difficult for people to understand how all-encompassing being a new mother is, and if you're struggling with postpartum depression, it's even more difficult to make time for your friends. Oftentimes PPD makes women retreat from their friends, because they don't want them to know something is wrong.

If you find yourself battling unrealistic expectations in any aspect of your life, you need to share your feelings with someone. You are not alone. There are people out there who do understand, have been there, and can help you be more realistic about your life.

Avoid Isolation

Depression has a way of turning people inward. When we're unhappy, it's often easier to stay at home, to stop talking to friends and family, than it is to be around other people. But isolating yourself will only make your postpartum depression worse. Making an effort to get out, to do things, and to talk to people may be difficult, but it's an essential part of your recovery. Talk with your partner, family, and friends about how you're feeling. Ask other mothers about their experiences. Ask your health-care practitioner about local support groups for new moms or women with postpartum depression. Talk to other mothers. You can learn from one another, and their experiences can be reassuring.

That said, there are also times when being alone is important and recommended. For instance, if you're exhausted from caring for your sick baby for the last few days, you really do need to have someone watch the baby while you stay in bed all day and sleep to recuperate.

This type of temporary isolation can help you heal and make you stronger. Just make sure to avoid constant isolation.

Limit Your Stressors

After the baby arrives, you may find that situations that were not stressful before have become big stressors for you now. This is a very sensitive time for you, and it's perfectly okay for you to set some limits in order to reduce the stress in your life. Here are some suggestions to help you keep from feeling too overloaded:

Don't make any major life decisions. The first several months after you've had your baby is not the time to make any big decisions. Significant life changes, such as moving to a new home, changing jobs, getting divorced, or having another baby (it's best to wait at least one year), have long-term consequences, and you'll be much better equipped to deal with these issues when your hormones have settled back into balance. This goes for your partner, too. Just because you're not making the big decision doesn't mean it won't have an impact on you. Encourage your partner not to change jobs or make big personal decisions until things have settled down at home. Joyce tells her patients to put any decisions that don't need to be made today on the back burner and let them simmer until they need to be discussed.

> *"I was planning an addition to my house while I was pregnant. Therapy helped me realize that waiting until after the baby was born would be a lot less stressful. Now that Patrick is here, it just doesn't seem as important. We've decided to put the addition off indefinitely."*
> —Laura G.

Keep phone calls short. It can be really stressful to hold a conversation on the phone and take care of your baby, especially if she's crying, so for the time being, don't even try. Let your machine pick up the call. Or if you get caught in a long conversation, tell the caller that you think you hear your baby crying and have to hang up. If possible, wait until your partner or a family member is there watching the baby before you return phone calls, and keep them short. Your free time is precious right now, so don't waste it all on the phone.

Set boundaries with friends and family. Once you're home with your new baby, your family and friends will want to come over to meet her, bring gifts, and see how you're both doing. Their hearts are in the right place, but having company over is work, and you need to focus on taking care of your baby and yourself right now. If you're feeling at all overloaded or stressed, say no to having visitors over. Just tell whoever wants to come over that you're tired and would prefer to do it another day, or have your partner tell her. She will understand. If you feel up to seeing people, that's great. But schedule visits in such a way that they don't interfere with your rest or otherwise stress you out. Plan visits at a time when your partner is home to help out, or if you're a single mom, ask a close friend or family member to come over to help you. If three of your friends have called and want to drop by, arrange for them all to come at the same time. Ask them to bring over lunch. Try to keep the visits short—we're not saying you should rush people out the door, but now probably isn't the best time to have people over for dinner and drinks.

SEVEN

Building Your Support System

A SOCIAL SUPPORT system is a network of family, friends, colleagues, and other acquaintances you can turn to, whether in times of crisis or simply for fun and entertainment. It is a powerful factor in every person's life, but especially so for women with postpartum depression. When going through a crisis like postpartum depression, it's not uncommon for women to withdraw from their partner, friends, and family and therefore not receive the support they so desperately need. Breaking through that isolation and reaching out for support may be one of the biggest obstacles you need to overcome, but it's a necessity. (This is particularly important for single moms, who do not have the benefit of a live-in partner to support them and are therefore inherently more isolated than women in a marriage or same-sex relationship.) Your recovery from postpartum depression depends on making sure you've got the support you need to see you through. In chapter 3 you read about how poor social support is a risk factor for PPD. In this chapter we talk about how crucial your social support system is to your treatment and your recovery from PPD and provide you with ideas for building and securing yours.

Finding the Right Support

Stress takes a big toll on your self-esteem and self-confidence, both of which you need in order to recover from postpartum depression. A good support system will nurture your self-esteem and self-confidence and relieve much of the stress in your life that's been weighing you down. Support systems can be big or small. Some people have big families, or like to surround themselves with many friends whom they can call on for help if necessary. Others prefer to have a smaller, more intimate group of people to count on. The size of your support system doesn't matter, as long as they are able to provide you with the types of help you need. Support usually comes from many different places and people. For instance, you may rely on your mother to come over and help you with the cleaning and the laundry, but maybe talking on the phone to your sister, who lives several states away, is what makes you smile. Or perhaps you don't count your next-door neighbor among your "good friends," but you know you can count on her to watch your baby for a few minutes while you run to the store. Sometimes just having another person in the house, not even interacting with you, can make you feel better.

It's equally important for you to eliminate from your support system anyone in your life who you feel will not be supportive. We're not telling you to cut these people out of your life entirely—just don't look to them for help, and try your best to limit the amount of time you spend with them while you're recovering. For example, if you don't get along with your mother-in-law, tactfully ask her not to visit for a week or so.

Support comes in various forms—financial, emotional, physical, educational, and practical, to name a few—and you may find that all of them will be helpful to you. It's rare to have one person in your life who can support you in every possible way; in fact, studies show that women with multiple sources of support adjust to the postpartum period more easily than women with a single source or none at all. So what you need to do is build yourself a system, or a team of people, who can provide you with all the kinds of support you need. It's a good idea to take some time to make a list of people and places that can offer you support. Writing it down might seem unnecessary, but since everyone has strengths and weaknesses, it will help you organize what person is best suited to support you in a particular way. The following are the best places to look for people for your support system.

Partner

Your partner is the person you are closest to, and therefore he is your most important source of support. In fact, studies show that if your partner is supportive during your pregnancy, labor, delivery, and the postpartum period, then you will be less likely to develop postpartum depression. When you have postpartum depression, a supportive partner will make your recovery faster and easier. We'll discuss how to get the support you need from your partner in chapter 9, so we won't go into detail here, but securing your partner's support should be at the top of your list. He is the person who can alleviate the most stress in your life. He may be the only person in your life in a position to help you on a daily basis. He can take on more responsibility around the house, give you a break from the baby every day, and be your shoulder to cry on in the middle of the night.

Family

After your partner, your family is probably the most important source of support in your life. You need to ask for and rely on the assistance of others during this time, and your family is there to take care of you. If you have a good relationship with your family or certain family members, it may be a lot easier for you to ask them for help than your friends or a health professional, because you trust and feel comfortable with them. You know that your family loves you unconditionally and that you can count on them to come through for you. It can be easier to ask family to handle chores like laundry and cleaning, and you may feel better about leaving your baby with your mother than with a friend or a babysitter. On the other hand, some women do not have a good relationship with their family, or find it difficult to tell their family about their postpartum depression, because they feel embarrassed or think that admitting they have PPD makes them too vulnerable. Some women feel comfortable telling only their mother and father, and not the rest of their family or their partner's family. It might be difficult, but we urge you to tell your entire family—the immediate and extended family on both your side and your partner's side—that you have postpartum depression. Many women are pleasantly surprised by how supportive their family can be, even the members with whom they don't have close relationships. Your family can be a huge resource for you, but they can't help you if they don't know you need help. You may need to educate them about your condition (see page 167 in chapter 9 about educating your partner on PPD for tips on doing this), but it's worth it.

Friends

Our friends are the people we confide in, depend on, and have fun with, and that's exactly the role they should play in your recovery from postpartum depression. It's easy to shut your friends out when you're going through a crisis—you may be afraid they'll be judgmental, or they won't understand, or perhaps you just don't have the energy or inclination to talk about your PPD. But think about how you would react if a friend in need came to you for help. Would you be judgmental? Would you refuse to help your friend because you didn't understand what she was going through? We doubt it. Your friends can offer all kinds of support as you work your way through PPD. They can listen when you want to talk. They can give you practical assistance, like driving you to a health-care practitioner's appointment or taking you to the store. They can come over and hang out with you when you're feeling alone. They can go for walks with you and the baby or be your exercise buddy. They can make you laugh. Different friends probably filled different needs for you before PPD, so think about which friend is best suited to fill each of your needs now. Who did you always call when you needed a laugh? Who was the best listener? Who would be the best person to call and ask for a ride? To babysit for an hour? Your friends want to be there for you—let them. It will have a huge impact on your recovery.

Neighbors

Your neighbors may not be the first people you think of when considering whom to include in your support system, but they can actually be very helpful to you during this time. You don't need to have a close or intimate relationship with someone to add him or her to your list of supporters. You only need to trust that person to support you in a specific or particular way. You may not have the type of relationship with your neighbor where you feel you can confide all of your feelings, but she may be the perfect person to watch your baby for an hour while you go to the store, take a walk by yourself, or take a much-needed nap. Your neighbor can help you make sure you have food in the house when you don't feel up to going out by picking up milk and other necessities for you when she goes to the grocery store for herself. If you have older children who are close in age to one of your neighbors' kids, she can have your kids over for a play date to give you a break. You can probably pay one of the neighborhood kids to help you with the upkeep of your house—he could mow your lawn, water your garden, or rake your leaves. Maybe one of your neighbors has a young son or daughter who's interested in being a mother's helper. A mother's helper is usually a girl age ten to thirteen or so who is too young to be left alone with a newborn but old enough to take some responsibility for the baby's care. Generally a mother's helper comes over for an hour or two after school a few days a week or at any time during her summer vacation. She can watch the baby while you nap or have some quiet time to yourself. She could feed the baby if you're not breast-feeding or if you've expressed milk for a bottle. A mother's helper may also be able to help you with some light housework duties and even some cooking. As an added bonus, you'll have a future babysitter who you and your baby know and trust.

Neighborhood mothers with young kids are also some of the best people to talk with and ask advice about babies. They're usually out in their yards or the street with the kids during the day in the warmer months, making them extremely easy to approach. More important, they can identify with much of what you're going through, regardless of whether they had postpartum depression themselves. They can also be great sounding boards for some of the problems you're facing and share some of their own hard-won advice with you.

Coworkers

If you've returned to the workplace, consider making some of your coworkers part of your support system. We're not saying you need to inform the entire office that you have postpartum depression, but telling a few trusted office friends can make your situation a lot easier and less stressful for you. Every job is different, but your coworkers may be in a position to help you with your work if you're feeling over-whelmed or unable to concentrate. If you work in a large enough office, chances are there are other women who've given birth recently or have young children who you could talk with and compare notes. They're probably feeling just as stressed and conflicted as you are about returning to work, and it's nice to be able to commiserate with others about it. Perhaps one of your coworkers would be interested in taking a walk with you at lunchtime each day to get a little exercise in.

Religious Communities

If you belong to a religious community, you are bound to find many different types of support there.

You can schedule time to talk with your religious leader about what you're going through. It can be a great relief to confide in an objective third party who you know will not judge you and will keep everything you say confidential. Your religious leader can also help you find ways to use your faith as a tool during your recovery.

Many religious organizations conduct women's groups that you could participate in. The groups may not be specifically for postpartum women, or even support groups of any nature, but getting together with other women might lift your spirits and make you feel more connected.

Some religious organizations have special groups that are trained through the church to provide one-on-one care to people who are facing life challenges or other difficulties. Their role is to listen and to care, not to give advice or counsel. Anything you tell them is strictly confidential. If you're looking for an impartial third party to talk with, you may find this type of arrangement suits you better than confiding in your religious leader.

You may also find that your church offers babysitting services, either on-site or at your home. If not, you can check the church bulletin board for people offering services such as babysitting and housecleaning.

Finally, many religious organizations have volunteers who visit people who are sick, disabled, or otherwise need help on a weekly basis and offer their services. You can add your name to your church's list and have the volunteer cook a meal for your family or help you tidy up the kitchen.

Professionals

You may want to include people in your support system who offer professional services that will help relieve some of your stress:

LACTATION CONSULTANT

Contrary to popular belief, breast-feeding can be difficult and arduous. It can take several weeks for you and your baby to get the hang of it, and many women have problems with pain, cracked nipples, latching-on issues, or fear that their baby isn't getting enough milk. If you are having problems but are determined to breast-feed, a lactation consultant can offer you some much-needed help in this area and set you on the right track. A lactation consultant will educate you on all aspects of breast-feeding, teach you new ways to position your baby to make you both more comfortable, solve latching-on problems, and help you feel more confident about breast-feeding in general.

Sue hired a lactation consultant after two weeks of what seemed like continuous breast-feeding, because she worried that she wasn't producing enough milk for her baby. The lactation consultant came to her house and talked with her for a while about her experience thus far and what she was feeling. She weighed Sue's baby and then gave him to Sue so that she could observe her breast-feeding and see if the baby was having trouble with latching on. She showed Sue several different ways to hold her baby while nursing, one of which allowed Sue to nurse while lying in bed, which was great for nighttime feedings. Together they worked out a schedule for nursing the baby and talked about how to deal with problems as they arose. The consultant also shared the experiences of other women she knew and had worked with, which made Sue feel a lot better. After Sue was finished with the breast-feeding session, the consultant weighed her baby again to show that he had indeed gotten a substantial amount of milk. She kept in touch with Sue in the weeks after her visit to answer questions and offer encouragement.

Lactation consultants can be expensive (Sue's cost $175 for a two-hour visit), but we think it's worth it if you are determined to make breast-feeding work. Finding one isn't too difficult—your obstetrician and your baby's pediatrician will probably have a few they can recommend, and the La Leche League can certainly recommend a consultant in your area. You can look up the La Leche League in your phone book, and you can also find them online at www.lalecheleague.org. (See Resources for further information on contacting the La Leche League.)

NANNY

A nanny is different from a babysitter in that she usually takes care of a family's child or children on a consistent basis. Typically people think of nannies as women who work full-time for one family for an extended period of time and live with them in their home. But nannies can actually be quite flexible—many are willing to work part-time, or full-time but not live with you, or full-time for a short period of time. They are usually expensive, but if you can afford it, a nanny can offer you a huge amount of help. She can aid you in every aspect of caring for your baby and give you a chance to rest and regain your strength. A live-in nanny can help you through the nights with your baby, taking over some or all of the feedings so that you can sleep. If you have older children, a nanny can help your children get off to school in the morning, greet them when they finish their school day, and bring them to practice and play dates. You'll be able to focus more of your energy on caring for your newborn and recovering from PPD.

BABY NURSE

Also known as a maternity nurse or a postpartum doula, a baby nurse is a newborn and infant care specialist. A baby nurse has extensive practical experience with newborns, as well as current knowledge of accepted practices in newborn care, including lactation support, Infant CPR certification, and the proper use of car seats. Many baby nurses also have some level of actual nursing training. The position of baby nurse is temporary in nature—generally two to eight weeks, though they often stay on longer in cases involving preemies and special needs infants. A baby nurse typically works twelve-hour shifts, either a day shift or a night shift, but often you can arrange for one to work a twenty-four-hour shift. A baby nurse's job is to provide you with assistance during the postdelivery recovery period and help you with all aspects of your baby's care, including feeding, changing, bathing, infant laundry, and helping you establish a schedule for your baby and get some much-needed rest.

According to www.nanniesandmore.com, wages for a baby nurse typically range between $20 and $30 per hour, or between $275 and $500 per day, depending on whether you're hiring her for a twelve-hour shift or a twenty-four-hour shift and if the care is for a single infant, twins, or triplets. In other words, a baby nurse is very expensive. But if you have the means, a baby nurse can be an immeasurable help to you.

HOUSEKEEPER

Another way to relieve some of your stress and get some practical support is to hire a housekeeper. When you have postpartum depression, taking care of yourself and your baby is essentially a full-time job. There isn't enough time or energy to spare to keep the house clean, do the laundry, and take care of all the other domestic chores that keep your household running smoothly. This can be a great source of stress for many women, particularly those who are used to being in control and doing what needs to be done around the house. Many women take great pride in keeping their homes looking clean and beautiful, and seeing dirty dishes, clothes strewn everywhere, and toys all over the floor just makes them feel even more overwhelmed and upset. Hiring a housekeeper to come over once or twice a week can help you stay on top of the domestic duties and free up time for you to focus on your recovery. A housekeeper will clean your home from top to bottom, make beds, and do your laundry and dishes. Some will even go grocery shopping and do other household-related errands for you. Housekeepers are relatively inexpensive—most typically earn between forty and sixty dollars per visit. You can hire one through a service like Molly Maid (www.mollymaid.com or 1-800-886-6559) or the Maid Brigade (www.maidbrigade.com), or you can look in your local paper for individuals who advertise their services. Often times you'll find flyers posted by people looking for cleaning jobs at your local YMCA, library, church, or community center.

> *"My mom's gift to me was hiring a housekeeper despite my protests. It was the best gift I received. I'm so glad she went ahead and did it!"*
>
> —Morgan F.

Hotlines

Most major hospitals have a telephone resource for women who have just given birth. This information will be given to you either at the hospital after the birth or possibly before by your health-care practitioner. Take advantage of these hotlines to speak with experienced counselors who will be able to offer you more than a shoulder to cry on. They can help you talk through your feelings and evaluate your situation to determine if you need to take further steps.

There are also some national hotlines you can call if you need to talk or if you want to locate support resources in your area, such as health-care professionals who specialize in postpartum depression, lactation consultants, support groups, and so on:

National Post Partum Depression Hotline: 800-PPD-MOMS
(773-6667).
PSI Postpartum Depression Helpline: 800-944-4773
Postpartum Depression Alliance Hotline: 847-205-4455

Internet Chat Rooms and Bulletin Boards

Sometimes it can be easier to ask questions or to look for support from the comfort and anonymity of your own home. That's where the Internet comes in. There are some fantastic support resources available on the Internet in the form of chat rooms and bulletin boards.

A chat room is a virtual room where people can communicate in real time while on the Internet. Users type their messages with a keyboard, and the entered text appears on the monitor, along with the text of the other chat room visitors. There are several sites that offer chat rooms devoted to postpartum depression. PPPSupportpage.com hosts three online PPD support groups each week.

Bulletin boards, also called newsgroups or discussion groups, work in a similar way to e-mail. Instead of writing messages to individual users, however, participants in bulletin boards post their messages on a news server. The messages are stored on the news server in hierarchical directories. Users participate in bulletin boards by reading the messages and responding to them.

Support Groups

A support group is a group of people all sharing a certain problem or concern who meet to discuss how they are dealing with it in a nurturing environment. One of the most difficult problems that new mothers face is handling the isolation they often feel after their babies are born. Many women feel like they're alone in dealing with the stresses of being a new mother. What support groups provide more than anything else is the opportunity to link up and feel a connection with other mothers. We strongly suggest you consider attending a support group as soon as you can after your baby is born. You may believe that you're not a "support group kind of person," that you need to focus your energy on other things right now, or that you don't have time for a support group, but joining one will make your postpartum period so much easier. Other new mothers know better than anyone else how you feel. There are two main types of support groups available for women adjusting to life with a new baby: new mother groups and postpartum depression support groups. You may want to try one of each type before deciding which one is best for you. Generally, women with mild cases of postpartum depression do well in new mother groups, while those with more severe cases of PPD find postpartum support groups more beneficial.

> *"Having a support system is a necessary and integral part of any woman's recovery from PPD."*
> —Joyce Venis

New mother groups are support groups formed to help new mothers meet and share their experiences. The members do not necessarily have postpartum depression, but they are usually experiencing some kind of trouble adjusting to life with a new baby. New mother support groups can be a great help, because they put you in the same room with women who've had babies at roughly the same time as you, so they understand at least some of what you are experiencing. They can also help you feel less isolated—hearing other women voice some of the fears and concerns that you may be having will show you that you are not alone in what you're going through and can make you feel more hopeful. You'll get to hear how other mothers deal with problems that you may be facing and go home with new ways of coping in your own life. You may even be able to help another new mother by sharing a tip or technique that's worked for you. Typically you bring your baby with you to a new mothers group, and many of them offer organized playtime for the babies.

There are also support groups available specifically for women with PPD. A postpartum depression support group is either led by a professional or by a woman who has recovered from her PPD and can offer her experience and knowledge to help other women recover. Unlike the new mothers support group, these groups are attended by women who suffer from some form of postpartum depression or anxiety, and the discussion is focused on coping with and recovering from the condition.

> *"Meeting with other women in the D.A.D. support group and sharing our experiences, successes, and feelings about PPD was an invaluable step toward my recovery. Now, as a coleader of a support group, I can give back to women suffering with PPD."*
>
> —Caroline R.

Both types of support groups usually meet once a week, though some may meet once a month. You don't have to talk unless you want to, and you can bring your kids to the meetings. There may be a fee to join the group, but if so it will be small.

A good place to start looking for a support group in your area is Postpartum Support International (PSI). This is a nonprofit organization dedicated to helping women who are experiencing perinatal mood disorders and providing them and their family members with information and referral services. You can call PSI at 800-944-4773, or visit their Web site at www.postpartum.net. Click on the "Support Groups and Area Coordinators" link on the menu and you'll find a list of support groups categorized by state. If there are no support groups listed in your area, contact your state's PSI coordinator for information on local resources. You can also contact your obstetrician or your baby's pediatrician—they should have information on what support groups are available in your area.

STARTING YOUR OWN SUPPORT GROUP

STARTING A support group for women with postpartum depression can be a very helpful and rewarding experience. If there is no support group that you can join in your area and you're interested in creating one, the following steps will help you get things moving.

1. Ask your health-care practitioner to tell other women with PPD that you are starting a group and where to contact you.

2. Write a simple press release announcing your intention to start a PPD support group and send it to your local paper, or take out a classified ad. We recommend that you don't include your phone number in the release or ad. Instead, rent a post office box for return mail. You could also post flyers announcing your intention to start a group at your library, community center, grocery store, and YMCA.

3. Choose a place to hold your meetings. You could have it in your own home or the home of another member of the group, but sometimes it's easier to talk freely in a neutral setting like a church, community center, or library.

4. Talk with the women who are interested in joining your group and set a date for meetings. You could meet once a week, once every two weeks, or once a month, depending on the group's needs and desires.

5. Your group doesn't need a permanent leader, but it's helpful to have one or two women set up and organize at least the first few meetings.

6. After several meetings, you may want to ask for a volunteer to lead the next week's meeting and choose a topic to discuss.

7. Make sure each woman has the opportunity to talk about her feelings.

8. Allow each woman to talk freely, openly, and without being judged.

9. Always stress the importance of confidentiality. No one will feel comfortable if she thinks what she says or does (even the fact that she's at a PPD support group meeting) could be discussed elsewhere.

10. Stress the importance of being proactive about their health and educating themselves on PPD by making materials such as brochures, books, and copies of magazine articles on PPD available to group members. You could collect donations at each meeting to subsidize these materials.

11. Supply the names of health-care practitioners who specialize in PPD and other perinatal mood disorders.

12. Invite health-care practitioners to speak at some of your meetings.

After you've established your PPD support group, you may decide you want to spread the word even further. You can inform all relevant local health-care professionals about your group and ask them to pass on your contact information (or designate someone else in the group as the contact person and give out her contact information) to any interested patients. You can ask these health-care professionals for permission to post a flyer in their waiting rooms. You can also place an ad or send a press release to your local newspaper with your meeting date, time, place, and name of your contact person.

If you're looking for more information on starting your own support group, there are two postpartum support organizations that offer help in forming and maintaining support groups on a local level:

Postpartum Support International
927 North Kellogg Ave.
Santa Barbara, CA 93111
Phone: 805-967-7636
Fax: 805-967-0608

National Association for Mothers' Centers (NAMC)
64 Division Ave.
Levittown, NY 11756
Phone: 800-645-3828

EIGHT

How PPD Affects Your Baby

BY NOW YOU know how important it is for you to seek treatment for postpartum depression as soon as possible. Women who reach out for help instead of "toughing it out" experience less severe symptoms and recover both faster and more completely. But here's another important reason why you need to address your postpartum depression quickly—you'll be safeguarding your baby's mental health.

Many studies have been done to try to determine what impact postpartum depression has on infant development. It has become quite clear that children whose mothers suffer from depression are at risk for developing many behavioral and learning problems. In other words, if you don't seek treatment for your postpartum depression, your baby could suffer consequences. The longer your child is exposed to untreated or mistreated postpartum depression, the more problems she could encounter.

What Do We Mean by Your Baby's "Mental Health?"

The term "infant mental health" describes both the social-emotional capacities and the primary relationships in children from birth through age five. Your child's social experiences and opportunities to explore the world depend on the love and care she receives, so both your child and her relationships are central to her mental health. It's essential to ensure that her first relationships are filled with trust and caring, because these early relationships provide an important foundation for her future development.

How Do Babies Develop Attachments?

Babies are hardwired to develop strong emotional connections with their primary caregivers. The ability to attach to a significant adult allows young children to become trusting, confident, and capable of dealing with stress and distress. The most important part of attachment is the quality of attachment formed, because it predicts later development.

Ideally, children develop secure attachment, or a healthy emotional bond, with their parents. Infants who develop secure attachment with their mother (or other primary caregiver) during the early years of life are more likely to have positive relationships with peers, be liked by their teachers, perform better in school, and respond with resilience in the face of adversity as preschoolers and older children. Attachment is integral to the emotional development of the young child; babies need to become attached to at least one close, trusting adult. In fact, a baby's need to attach is so strong that he will even develop an emotional connection with inconsistent and insensitive caregivers if the right kind of care is unavailable. Infants who develop insecure attachment are at risk of developing learning delays, relationship dysfunction, difficulty expressing emotions, and future mental health disorders.

How PPD Can Affect Your Parenting

Studies have shown that postpartum depression can have an affect on your ability to parent. Here are the key reasons why:

You're at risk for providing inconsistent care. Studies show that postpartum depression may cause mothers to be inconsistent with child care. When you're depressed, you may not respond as quickly or as positively to your baby's cues as you need to. If your depression is severe, you may not be able to respond to your baby at all. This can affect the development of a secure bond between the two of you. If you don't respond to your baby consistently in a warm, caring way—holding, rocking, cooing, stroking, or talking softly—your baby may have trouble feeling safe, secure, and trusting. If your baby feels insecure, he may have trouble interacting with you.

PPD can create an unhealthy environment. When you're depressed, you're less social, friendly, and enthusiastic than usual. You're more likely to express negative words and emotions than positive ones. Your tone of voice may also be affected. Depression can cause your voice to become flat and unexpressive. A recent study looked at 225 four-month-old infants, and their responses to the voices of depressed and nondepressed women. Babies do not learn as well when they are listening to the flatter, less melodic voices of depressed women. An adult's perky, high-pitched baby talk sets the stage for intellectual development. In order to create a healthy environment for your baby, you need to play with her, talk to her, cuddle with her, and generally provide a lot of positive stimulation. Postpartum depression can make this difficult or even impossible.

PPD may affect how you perceive your baby. Mothers with postpartum depression are more likely to express negative attitudes about their baby and to view their baby as more demanding or difficult. Depressed mothers also often have difficulty engaging their baby. They're either more withdrawn than they should be or inappropriately intrusive. To be inappropriately intrusive means you're *too* involved with your baby or you're overstimulating her.

Likewise, your baby's personality can influence the way you respond to him. Studies show that a child who elicits negative or minimal interactions with his depressed mother may cause her to feel rejected and further discourage her efforts to develop mother-child intimacy. Depressed mothers' perceptions that their infants are more difficult may actually be correct. This sets up a challenging dynamic, where neither mother nor child has positive experiences with or expectations of the other.

> *"When I had a very bad day, my baby would have a bad night. There seemed to be a pattern. Once I got appropriate treatment, including therapy, this dynamic changed greatly. We're much closer now than I ever imagined after what I went through."*
>
> —Francine G.

BABY'S INTUITION

INFANTS ARE highly sensitive to a mother's sadness, silence, and inattentiveness. In one study, mothers of three-month-old infants were asked to simulate depression for three minutes. They spoke in a monotone, remained expressionless, and avoided touching the child. Even at that age infants could respond to brief changes in their mothers' apparent mood. They looked away from their mothers and showed signs of distress, which continued for a while even after the women began to behave normally.

> *"I'm grateful for having had PPD and for what I went through, because I have a much stronger and healthier*

relationship with my daughters now. I feel I'm a better mother now than I was then."

—Barb M.

How PPD Can Affect Babies

The first years of life provide the basis for your baby's mental health and social-emotional development. Social development includes both the ability to form healthy relationships with others and the knowledge of social rules and standards. Emotional development includes the experience of feelings about self and others, with a range of positive and negative emotions, as well as the ability to control and regulate feelings in culturally appropriate ways. The development of self-worth, self-confidence, and self-regulation are important features of social-emotional development. Healthy social-emotional development is essential for success in school and in life. Here are the key ways untreated postpartum depression can affect infants:

They may become negative. A baby is typically in tune with the emotional signals in his mother's voice, gestures, movements, and facial expressions. As a result, young children whose mothers are depressed display more negative and less positive emotions than those children who have nondepressed mothers.

They may become chronically irritable. Your baby may also be more irritable, difficult to soothe, and less "happy." Children of depressed mothers often learn from the patterns of their early experiences and perceive that only negative strategies, such as fussing or crying, will elicit a response. Unfortunately, such negative expectations often become the child's standard way to seek attention.

They may reject their mothers. Babies of depressed mothers often reject them or become upset with them in response to a lack of positive interaction or inability to meet her needs.

They may develop behavioral problems. Children of mothers with untreated postpartum depression are more likely than children of nondepressed mothers to exhibit anxiety and behavioral problems, such as sleep and eating difficulties, temper tantrums, and hyperactivity.

They may experience delayed development. Evidence suggests that children with depressed mothers may experience developmental delays, meaning they don't reach milestones as quickly as they should. Developmental milestones are a set of functional skills or age-specific tasks that most children can do at a certain age range. Your pediatrician uses milestones to help gauge how your child is developing. Although each milestone has an age level, the actual age when a normally developing child reaches that milestone can vary quite a bit, as every child is unique.

They may develop emotional disorders. Infants and toddlers of depressed mothers can develop serious emotional disorders, such as infant depression and attachment disorders. Early mental health disorders might be reflected in overall delayed development, inconsolable crying, or sleep problems.

They may have language problems. Maternal depression reduces consistent and readable communication between mother and child, and as a result poor language development may occur, with vocabulary deficits still present at early school age.

They may be susceptible to illness. Children of depressed mothers see their primary care physicians more often and have higher rates of prescription medications and hospitalizations than children of nondepressed mothers.

They may act withdrawn. Kids with depressed mothers often become withdrawn and passive. Studies show that infants of clinically depressed mothers often withdraw from daily activities and avoid interaction with caregivers, which in turn jeopardizes infant language and physical, emotional, and intellectual development.

They may act depressed. Evidence of infants experiencing symptoms of depression has been found in children as young as four months old.

The Effects Can Be Long-Lasting

Studies also reveal that untreated or mistreated postpartum depression may have long-lasting effects. Older children of mothers who were depressed during the child's infancy show poor self-control, aggressive or impulsive behavior, poor peer relationships, and difficulty in school. In early care and education settings, children with social and emotional problems tend to have a difficult time relating to others, trusting adults, being motivated to learn, and calming themselves to tune into teaching—all skills that are necessary to benefit from early educational experiences.

Older children may also develop attachment issues. They may be less independent and less likely to interact with other people. They may have discipline, behavior, and aggression issues. Some children with these issues have a higher risk of mental health issues, such as anxiety and depression. Children of depressed parents in general are highly vulnerable to depression, and long-term adjustment is sometimes also a problem.

Minimizing Your Baby's Risks

You're probably a little nervous now after reading about all the ways untreated or mistreated postpartum depression might affect your relationship with your baby and her mental health. Clearly, having PPD puts your baby at risk, especially if you don't seek treatment. But there are ways that you can counteract the effect PPD may have on your little one. We have listed some of them below, but it's important to note that the most important step you can take to minimize your baby's risks is to get treatment for your PPD. Although few studies have examined the ways treatment affects the mother–infant relationship, evidence has shown that treatment will significantly improve both your mood and the quality of your relationship with your baby.

Talk to your baby. One of the best ways you can interact with your baby and keep her stimulated is to talk to her. It doesn't really matter what you say, just as long as you're making an effort to connect with her. She may not understand what you're saying yet, but she's definitely listening. Here are some tips for talking to your baby:

- Look at your baby's eyes while you're talking to her.
- Call your baby by her name.
- Narrate a task that you're performing, like changing her diaper or getting her dressed. Tell her why you're doing it and what you're thinking.
- Keep your talk simple, and refer to yourself as "Mommy" when you're talking about yourself. "Mommy's going to give you a bath now."
- Watch your baby's expressions and listen to her sounds. Make these same sounds and facial expressions back to her.
- Add gestures to your talk. Say, "Wave bye-bye to the dog" as you wave to the dog.
- Ask your baby questions even though she can't answer yet. "Would Lisa like to have her milk now?" "Does Lisa want to go outside?"
- Sing to your baby. You can sing her old children's songs, like "Mary Had a Little Lamb," or your favorite rock songs— she'll love anything you sing. (If you've forgotten the words to those old children's songs, do a search online for children's

songs or lyrics. A good place to start is Parenting Universe, at www.parentinguniverse.com/Songs/SongsMain.html.)

Source: U.S. Department of Agriculture, U.S. Department of Education and U.S. Department of Health and Human Services, *Healthy Start, Grow Smart: Your Two-Month-Old,* Washington, DC, 2002.

Read to your baby. It's never too early to start reading to your baby. Books are a great way to entertain your baby and build a relationship with her in the first months of her life. Babies learn that reading is important when you hold them, show them pictures in a book, and talk about the pictures. They enjoy being read to, because they like the sound of your voice and having you close for some special time together. Babies enjoy looking at the pictures and listening to the rhythm of your voice long before they can understand the words. Reading to your baby encourages the development of a range of important skills, such as talking and understanding language, imagination, concentration, creativity, listening, and problem solving. Children whose parents read books to them when they are young often learn to speak, read, and write more easily.

Between the ages of six months and one year, a board book's hard, chewable cover is perfect for small hands and a baby's attention. When you're reading, try to bring the story to life. Make faces and sounds, point to pictures, ask questions, and talk about what you and your baby are seeing on the pages.

Babies love to hear the same words again and again. Capture their interest with *Goodnight Moon* by Margaret Wise Brown and Clement Hurd, *The Very Hungry Caterpillar* by Eric Carle, or other stories where your child can guess what happens next. When your baby starts talking, she'll love the fact that she knows the story well enough to repeat words or chant along with the story.

STORY TIME

READING TO your baby will not only strengthen your bond, but it will also instill in her a love of books that will last a lifetime. Here are a few classic board books that we think you and your baby will enjoy:

Goodnight Moon by Margaret Wise Brown and Clement Hurd

The Big Red Barn by Margaret Wise Brown and Clement Hurd

The Very Hungry Caterpillar by Eric Carle

Brown Bear, Brown Bear, What Do You See? by Eric Carle and Bill Martin

Ten Little Ladybugs by Melanie Gerth

The Rainbow Fish by Marcus Pfister

Belly Button Book by Sandra Boynton

How Do Dinosaurs Clean Their Room? by Jane Yolen and Mark Teague

How Do Dinosaurs Count to Ten? by Jane Yolen and Mark Teague

Oops! by David Shannon

Oh David! by David Shannon

Make an effort to play. Playing is another great way to create and support attachment, communication, and caring between you and your child. Baby's play is also a very important part of his development—it fosters physical, intellectual, emotional, and social skills. In addition, it's an important factor in the formation of his identity and personality.

When you're depressed, playing might be the last thing you want to do, but it will truly do both you and your baby a world of good. Interacting with your baby, getting down on his level, being silly to make him smile—all of these things can help brighten your mood as well as entertain and stimulate your baby. And once you get started, you'll see it's easier to muster the energy and enthusiasm than you thought it would be. If you're not sure where to start, here are some ideas for different ways you can engage in play:

- **Play peek-a-boo.** Babies love to play peek-a-boo. You can play the traditional way, by hiding your face behind your hands, or you can hide yourself just out of your baby's line of sight and pop up to get a laugh.
- **Get down on the floor with your baby.** You are your child's ultimate plaything, and any activity will seem more fun if your baby can share it with you. Babies also need time on their tummies to learn how to push up and eventually crawl. Get down on your tummy with him and show him how his rattle works, or how soft his stuffed animal is.
- **Make bath time fun.** If you're still bathing your baby in a baby tub, make a game out of it. Wiggle his legs while you're washing them, or clap his hands together so he can see the water splash. Once your baby graduates from his baby tub, you can make bath time even more fun. Buy a set of cups especially made for the bath or some of those plastic creatures that squirt water, and show him how they work. There are many bath toys available that your baby will find interesting.
- **Take your baby outside.** Your baby will find the outdoors endlessly interesting—there's so much to see! Take your baby to the park and set up camp on a bench or on the grass. Position him so that he can see as much as possible, and let him drink it all in. Point out the trees, the leaves, the flowers, the birds, the other kids, and talk about them. What color are the flowers? What kind of birds are they? Or you and your baby can simply sit together in your backyard. Let him feel the grass. Place him on a blanket and let him look at the clouds. Bring a ball out with you and roll it back and forth with him. Or buy a splash pool and sit in it with him. Babies usually love the water, and it's a great way to keep cool in the summer months. You could also go to your local playground and watch the older kids play while you describe what they're doing. Babies are fascinated

with other children. If your baby is old enough (usually about the time they're able to stand), he may enjoy being pushed on the infant swings or going down the slide with you. You could take your baby for a walk into town so that he can see the stores and the cars.

NINE

How PPD Affects
Your Relationship
with Your Partner

HAVING A BABY is a stressful event for every couple. In fact, studies show that marital conflict and dissatisfaction are very common in the first year after childbirth. But when you have postpartum depression, those "normal" stresses and pressures that every couple must deal with can become dramatically worse.

Whether this is your first baby or your fourth, as a new mother you need your partner's support while you adjust to life with your baby. When you have postpartum depression, that need increases a hundredfold. This chapter will help you find ways to meet your need for support, and also help you understand your partner's perspective and what he is going through as a result of your condition. (As we mentioned in the introduction, for the sake of convenience, we refer to your partner as a "he," but the information also applies to female partners.)

Your Partner's Perspective

Chances are that your partner is just as confused by what you're going through as you were before you began to educate yourself on postpartum depression. He certainly never expected you would react this way after the baby was born, and he probably has no idea what to do for you. Your partner is also going through an adjustment period of his own with a new baby in the house, and he still has to go to work every day. Now he has to take on many of your responsibilities, because you're unable to meet them right now. He doesn't understand what's going on, or why, and there doesn't seem to be an end to the situation in sight. That's not to say that your partner doesn't want to help you—most men try their best to help their partner cope with what they're going through. But there's no denying that living with postpartum depression is stressful and difficult for your partner, and there are a range of reactions and emotions that he may experience. Most partners go through a mix of the reactions we list below.

Anger

Some men react to their partner's postpartum depression with anger. They're angry that you feel the way you do. They're angry that your condition is making life so difficult for everyone. They don't understand what you're going through and why you can't just snap out of it. They may even blame you for your illness, believing you did something to cause it. They're angry that they have to pick up the slack for you around the house and with the baby in addition to their other responsibilities. Some men become angry because their expectations have gone unrealized. Life with baby has not turned out the way they expected or wanted it to so far.

> "My wife was so angry about everything. I was angry, too, . . . at people for saying this was supposed to be the best time of my life. It wasn't."
>
> —Dave Z.

Depression

Other men become caught up in the emotions you're feeling and start feeling down and anxious themselves. In fact, studies show that nearly one third of women who have postpartum depression have a depressed partner. It's easy to see how your partner could start feeling depressed when he's living with someone who's feeling sad, crying all the time, having mood swings, and so forth. In addition, many men are not sure how to take care of babies. We've already explained that parenting is a learned skill, but many fathers hold the old-school notion that their job is to earn the money and play with their kids, not to feed, diaper, and bathe them. They've not given a second thought to what is involved in caring for an infant and are usually even more unprepared for it than new mothers are. They also often feel overwhelmed by the added responsibilities they've had to take on in order to keep everyday life running somewhat smoothly.

Frustration

Some men become frustrated with their partner because she has postpartum depression. They don't understand what you're going through, and they think your moods and feeling are in your control. Many men start out being sympathetic to their partner's condition but grow increasingly irritated when the situation doesn't get better. They also feel helpless because nothing they do or say makes you feel better and they don't know how to help you. Some get frustrated because they feel like they've gotten a raw deal. Their partner has PPD, so they have to work extra hard to take care of everything around the house. They often don't understand that you are simply incapable of doing a lot right now. They wonder why this is happening to them and their family.

> *"Stan comes home from work and expects to be able to read the paper. He gets so frustrated when I ask him to help me out by giving the baby a bath or a bottle, as if his day should be over when he comes home from work."*
> —Betty J.

Fear

Postpartum depression can be scary for your partner. Unless you have a history of depression or anxiety, he's probably not accustomed to seeing you like this. He's worried about your health. He's worried about the baby. He's not sure what to do—will this go away on its own? Should he get you help? Who should he turn to? He also may be scared because he's not sure when or even if your depression will end. He's afraid you may never return to your old self and feels like he's lost his best friend and partner.

Abuse

If there is a history of abuse in your relationship with your partner, it will most likely continue and may even intensify in response to your postpartum depression. Your partner is under enormous stress right now with you unwell and a new baby to care for. If he has a propensity for physically or verbally abusing you, the circumstances are right for a meltdown. If this happens, our advice is to take your baby and leave. We know this is easier said than done, but it's important to your health and to your baby's well-being that you remove yourself from an abusive situation. Go stay at your parents' house for a while, or at a good friend's house, until things cool down and you can figure out your next move.

Even some men who have no history of abuse have been known to snap and say nasty, verbally abusive things to hurt their partner. If your partner has uncharacteristically behaved in this manner, we advise that you bring your partner with you to your PPD therapist to try to resolve the issue.

Although typically it's assumed that men are the abusers, it's not uncommon for women to become abusive during their PPD. Lindsay K. pulled a knife on her partner after he told her to "get a grip" on her emotions. If your situation is getting volatile, remove yourself from it and call your therapist.

How to Get the Support You Need

Having your partner's full support is a key component in your recovery. Although your partner may not be acting the way you hoped he would or need him to right now, rest assured that he does want to help you get through your depression and return to your old self. He just needs a little help from you to accomplish this. Here are some steps you can take to help your partner give you the support you need:

1. **Educate him.**

   As we mentioned earlier, your partner most likely has no idea what postpartum depression is and how it's affecting you. You need to explain it to him. Ask him to read chapter 1 of this book, or sit down with him and describe the condition yourself. Either way, there are a few key points that you should make sure he understands:

   - Postpartum depression is a mood disorder that is triggered by the act of giving birth. It affects up to 20 percent of new mothers and is considered the most common complication of childbirth.
   - A combination of biological, psychological, and social factors have caused you to suffer from it. In other words, it is not your fault you have PPD, and you are not generating these symptoms yourself.
   - Postpartum depression is a very treatable condition. With therapy, medication, and his support, your condition will get better and you will return to your old self soon.

   It can also be very helpful to bring your partner with you to your PPD support group meetings. He'll learn a lot about the condition and will understand that you are by no means alone in what you're going through.

2. **Communicate your needs clearly.**

   Good communication is important to every relationship— baby or no baby. After you and your partner had been together for a while, you probably developed your own way of communicating, using a combination of verbal and nonverbal communication. Verbal communication is pretty clear—you share your thoughts and feelings with each other, and you talk out your issues. Nonverbal communication is a little more subtle. It's the way we communicate with one another using our bodies, with gestures, touching, eye contact, and facial expressions. For instance, stroking your partner's arm in bed could be a signal for sex that is simply understood between the two of you. Or the pile of newspaper by the door is a signal for the person leaving to take it out and toss it in the recycling bin.

Both verbal and nonverbal communication are good, healthy ways to express yourself. But when you have postpartum depression, it becomes vitally important for you to communicate your feelings and needs clearly, and nonverbal communication can be easily misinterpreted in times of stress. You may believe, based on your partner's actions, that he's frustrated with you, uninterested in what you're feeling, or disappointed in you, when in reality that's not how he feels. Your partner may believe that you're angry with him, you think he never does anything right, or you blame him for what's going on, when you don't think that at all. This type of constant miscommunication can be very damaging to your relationship, because it will drive the two of you further and further apart. You'll wind up feeling even more alone and unsupported, which will make coping with postpartum depression all the more difficult. This might sound silly, but you need to remind yourself every day that your partner cannot read your mind. You have to make a concerted effort to *talk* with him about how you feel and what you need. You should even do this during those times when you don't know what you want or need. Simply telling him that you're not sure how you feel or what you need may be enough to clear the air.

Good communication is all in the approach. Your goal here is to tell your partner what you need from him to make things better and let him know how he can best support you while you work through your postpartum depression. Here are some tips for communicating your needs in the most productive way:

- **Use "I" statements.** The last thing you want to do is to sound accusatory. Your partner will probably become defensive or feel like you expect him to know how you feel and what he should do at all times. Instead of saying, "Why do you always have to come home so late from work?" try saying, "I could really use a little time to myself after a long day with the baby. Could you possibly come home early from work once or twice a week so I can have a break?" This way you're explaining what you need and why in a calm and open way.

  Another effective communication technique is to follow the pattern "I feel _____ when you do _____." For instance, you could say, "I feel like you think I'm stupid when you constantly tell me how to do things."

- **Be specific.** Telling your partner exactly what you need will ensure that your need gets met. Saying, "Why do you always have to come home so late from work?" doesn't necessarily translate to "I really need a break" for your partner. Don't be afraid to express what you want.

  Making an effort to be specific is good for you in another way. Sometimes you may not be sure what you need. Your thoughts are jumbled, and all you know is that you're not happy and that your partner is not helping matters. You can't ask for support until you know what kind of support you need. Thinking about what you want to ask of your partner can help you distinguish what you actually do need.

- **Ask him to clarify.** Your perception of what your partner means when he says or does something could be completely wrong, so always ask for clarification. For example, if you have plans to meet your partner for lunch and he calls to cancel without giving a reason, ask him to explain. This way you'll know that he can't meet you because he has to attend an important meeting instead of assuming that he doesn't want to spend time with you because you're always feeling down.

- **Make rules.** Lay down some communication ground rules that you both agree to follow. There should be no name-calling or yelling at each other. Allow each other to speak without interruption. Always resolve whatever issue you are discussing before parting ways. Don't stockpile your issues—address problems and concerns as they arise.

- **Be empathetic.** Do your best to look at what's happening from your partner's point of view and to accept his emotions, thoughts, and feelings. It's not always easy to do this, since PPD tends to make you focus on yourself and not on others, but showing some empathy for what your partner is going through will score a lot of points with him. It will also make communication a lot easier and free-flowing, and it will show your partner how much you care about him.

3. **Be open about how PPD is affecting you.**

   You've already educated your partner about postpartum depression in general, and now you need to help him understand how it's affecting you personally. Try to be as open and honest about your symptoms as you can. Explain to him as clearly as possible what your symptoms are, how they make you feel, and what you believe may trigger them. If possible, point out a particular symptom as it's happening. For instance, perhaps your baby is screaming and won't go to sleep, and you're feeling very stressed and upset about it. You know from experience that this situation may very well trigger a panic attack for you, and you're beginning to feel those familiar sensations that tell you one is brewing now. Tell your partner that you're feeling a little panicky. Sometimes all you need to quell those panicky feelings is for him to give you a hug and tell you everything will be fine. It will also give your partner a very clear picture of what types of situations may be difficult for you right now, and he'll be more apt to act supportive when you find yourselves there again.

You should also try to be as open as you can with your partner about your perception of things. Your PPD is certainly coloring your view of your life, your baby, and your relationship with your partner, family, and friends. Talk with him about your views. If you can, explain why you believe you see things in a particular way. Doing so will give your partner a chance to put himself in your shoes and better understand what you're going through.

4. **Offer your partner concrete ways to help you.**
   Oftentimes your partner may want to help you, but he doesn't know what to do. Give him some tangible ways that he can offer support and make your life easier. Really think about this and make a list of ideas. Your goal is to alleviate some of your stress, so no task is out of bounds. You should include everything from housework to entertainment. If you think he might appreciate it, share the list with him so that he can see what you would find helpful and supportive. Or you can keep it to yourself and simply tell him what you need when you need it. Here are some ideas:

- Do a load of laundry
- Cook dinner
- Clean up the kitchen
- Give the baby her nighttime feeding
- Take the baby for a walk while you rest
- Answer the phone and tell callers that you're sleeping
- Do the grocery shopping
- Rent a movie for you to watch
- Give the baby her bath
- Take you and the baby for a drive
- Watch the baby while you go get a pedicure
- Get up early a few mornings a week with the baby so you can get some extra sleep

5. **Make him part of your treatment.**
   Your partner plays a significant role in your recovery from postpartum depression. His support will help you get better

faster and more easily. His lack of support will make the recovery process slower and more difficult for you. A great way to secure your partner's support is to keep him in the loop and make him an active participant in the treatment process. Here are some ways you can do this:

Bring your partner to your appointments with your health-care practitioner. Bringing your partner with you accomplishes three important things. First, it keeps him completely up-to-date on how you're feeling, the progress you're making, and what your health-care practitioner has to say. It will help your partner feel involved in your recovery in a very special way. You also won't need to rehash what happened and what was said at every appointment, because he'll be there with you. Second, participating in your appointments will educate your partner even further on postpartum depression. He'll have the chance to ask questions and get professional answers. Finally, having your partner along at your appointments gives your health-care practitioner another perspective on your symptoms and recovery. It's not unusual for your partner to observe things in you that you are not aware of, and this knowledge can be extremely helpful to your health-care practitioner.

Ask for his opinion. Ultimately, you need to make your own decisions about your treatment and what's best for you. But asking for your partner's opinion on issues can be very beneficial. It will make him feel like he's participating in your recovery. It will give you another perspective on every decision you must make. And talking an issue through with someone you love and trust, weighing the pros and cons together, can help you make the best possible decisions.

Talk about your therapy sessions. Therapy sessions can be intense, emotional, and thought provoking. Not every woman is comfortable sharing what goes on in her therapy sessions with her partner, and that's perfectly fine. Keep what goes on in therapy private if you have any reservations about discussing it. But if you're open to the idea, we suggest sharing some or all of what goes on in therapy with your partner. It can help crystallize concepts you may be wrestling with, and it's another way to include your partner in the treatment process.

We also suggest you take your partner with you to some of your therapy sessions so that he can ask questions and offer input that your therapist may find very valuable.

6. **Create "couple time."**

Usually the first sacrifice a new mother must make after her baby arrives is time with her partner. New mothers tend to focus most of their attention on taking care of their babies, which leaves little room for anything else in their lives. But if you neglect your relationship with your partner, you may begin to feel emotionally disconnected from each other, which makes it a lot more difficult for you to ask for the support you need and for him to give it. We know this is a lot easier said than done, but it's crucial that you spend time together as a couple, just the two of you. Spending time together is the best way to remain close and maintain your bond. You need to make time and steal time whenever you can. You don't necessarily need to spend the entire time talking—just being together is therapeutic. When you do talk, try to steer the conversation away from the baby. Talk about your partner's job, or what your friends have been doing, or how your sister is. You could also talk about special moments from your past, such as how you and your partner met or good times you've had together. Reminiscing about your shared history will make you feel closer to one another. Of course it's fine to talk about the baby and even your postpartum depression if you need to, but try not to make it the focus of your time together. Remember, you're doing this to strengthen your bond. Your relationship with your partner will continue to grow and change, and you both need to work at nurturing it. Do your best to enjoy the precious little time you have together alone. Here are some ideas for creating "couple time":

- It will do you a world of good to get out of the house together, even for an hour or two. Create a standing date once every two weeks (once a week would be even better) when someone comes over to babysit and the two of you go out. Go to dinner, take a walk, see a movie—just make sure you leave the house for a while.
- Conversely, have someone come over and take your baby out while you and your partner spend some alone time at home.
- Drop your baby off at your mom's and have your partner play hooky from work for a day.
- Order takeout from your favorite restaurant and eat together after the baby goes to bed.
- Have your partner rent a new movie that you've been wanting to see, then watch it together while your baby naps.
- When you get into bed at night, ask your partner to come in and lie down with you for a few minutes. He doesn't necessarily need to rub your back (although that would be very nice), but you should make an effort to snuggle up together while you drift off to sleep or watch TV.
- If your partner works nearby, he might be able to come home when the baby is napping to spend some alone time with you once or twice a week.
- If your baby takes a late afternoon/early evening nap, ask your partner to come home from work early once or twice a week so that you can have some quiet time together before she wakes up.

7. **Spend time together with your baby.**

Spending time together as a family is important for many reasons. As we described in chapter 8, your baby is hardwired to develop an emotional attachment to his primary caregivers. This attachment, or bond, begins to form in the first days of your baby's life and is accomplished when you respond to your baby consistently in a warm, caring way—holding, rocking, cooing, stroking, or talking softly to him. Spending time together as a family will strengthen and perpetuate that bond with both you and your partner. It also gives you the chance to watch your baby grow together. It's a very rewarding bonding experience when the two of you together see your baby do something new, like smile, babble, or show an interest in something.

Many men have no idea how to care for a baby. Giving him a bath, changing his diaper, or putting him down for a nap together will not only relieve some of your stress, but it will also show your partner how to attend to your baby's needs so that he can begin doing so on his own. Here are some other activities that you and your partner could do together with your baby:

- Snuggle on the couch for bedtime stories, and take turns reading pages with your partner.
- Get down on the floor and play some games with her. You could roll a ball between the three of you, or show him how to stack blocks—any kind of play will do.
- Strap your baby into his stroller and go for a walk. Or pack a simple picnic lunch and spend an hour at the park together.
- Join a class together. There are many types of classes that the three of you can participate in as a family. Wellness centers, hospitals, community centers, and YMCAs offer everything from educational parenting classes to baby gymnastics classes to infant massage classes. Check your local Yellow Pages and call the centers nearest you to see what they offer.

Sex

Sex is almost always an issue for women after giving birth to a baby, regardless of whether or not they have postpartum depression. Your body needs time to recover from the physical demands of childbirth—Caesarean section incisions, perineal tearing, episiotomy stitches, and general soreness all play a role. You may also be contending with the demands of breast-feeding, and most certainly with exhaustion and hormone changes. Emotionally you may be feeling self-conscious, unattractive, or overweight. You might be afraid of getting pregnant again. All of these factors can contribute to a loss of sex drive. Postpartum depression makes a loss of sex drive even more likely, since extreme fatigue, low self-esteem, and body image issues usually go hand in hand with PPD. Another factor that may be influencing your sex drive is medication. If your health-care practitioner has put you on an antidepressant to help combat your postpartum depression, it's possible that your loss of libido is a side effect of the medication. (See chapter 5 for advice on counteracting sexual side effects.) The bottom line is that losing your sex drive is completely normal given your situation, and it's a temporary condition. Try your best not to feel guilty about it.

Talking about sex with your partner may be difficult and uncomfortable for you even in the best of times, but right now it's a necessity. Your partner probably doesn't understand why you're not interested in sex. Most men count the days until the obstetrician has given their partner the green light to resume sex. Many think they can just pick up their sex life where they left off before the baby was born. You need to communicate with your partner and explain that your lack of interest in sex is one of the symptoms of postpartum depression and assure him that your desire will return. Tell him that this is a temporary condition. Make sure he understands that it was not caused by problems in your relationship and that he shouldn't take it personally. If you find that talking to your partner face-to-face is just too difficult, you can write him a note explaining all of this. You can also take him to some of your therapy sessions so that you can address the issue together with the help of a professional. What's most important is that you are both on the same page about your sex life.

You also need to let your partner know the kind of intimacy that you *do* need right now. Many women find that they have an increased need for cuddling and touching while working through their PPD. If you don't verbalize this, your partner may mistake this need for a sexual advance, which will put you both in an unhappy position. One way to encourage your partner to be affectionate with you is to reinforce the behaviors you like, by saying things like, "I love it when you stroke my hair." Or, "When we hold hands while we're watching television, I realize you love me even though I'm not ready for sex." You could also ask for nonsexual massages or foot rubs. Your partner should know that you appreciate his touch outside of lovemaking, and that a kiss on the back of your neck while you're tending to your baby sends shivers (the good kind) down your spine.

TEN

When Your Loved One Has Postpartum Depression

WHEN A WOMAN has postpartum depression, her illness affects everyone around her. As her partner, family, and friends, it can be very difficult for you to cope with what she's going through and its impact on you. You may not understand what's going on, why this is happening to her, or what you can to do to help. You may be going through a tough time yourself—this baby has changed your lives, too, and you probably have had to take on many of the tasks and duties that your loved one can't handle right now. This chapter is designed to offer you information, support, and coping mechanisms for living with someone who has postpartum depression. It will also show you how you can best support her as she works to recover from her illness.

Understanding Postpartum Depression

When your loved one is diagnosed with postpartum depression, one of the first things you should do is educate yourself about this disorder. You need to understand the nature of the illness your loved one has in order to handle its effect on you and to support her through her recovery. In fact, the more you understand what she is going through, the more supported she will feel. This, in turn, will help her recover faster.

Postpartum depression is a very real and serious mood disorder. It's difficult to give a simple explanation of the disorder because of its rather complex nature, but postpartum depression is generally defined as a state of persistent sadness or anxiety that lasts longer than two weeks after childbirth. The exact cause of postpartum depression is unknown, but most experts agree that it is triggered by a combination of biological, sociological, and psychological factors after the birth of a baby. It is not your loved one's fault that she has postpartum depression—the circumstances of her life interacted in such a way as to give her PPD. There is nothing that she, you, or anyone else did to cause this to happen. There is also nothing that you can do to "fix" things for her. Recovering from postpartum depression takes time and professional help. What she needs from you is your complete support while she's going through this.

When some people hear the phrase "postpartum depression," they associate it with the news stories they've heard about women doing crazy things or harming their children, like the story of Andrea Yates, who drowned her five children in the bathtub in 2001. It's important for you to understand that these women suffer from postpartum psychosis, which is a type of postpartum mood disorder that is different from and more severe than what your loved one is suffering from. Women with postpartum depression sometimes have thoughts about hurting their children (these are called intrusive thoughts and are symptoms of the illness), but they *never* act on them. You don't need to worry about her baby's physical safety.

Postpartum depression is more common than you may think. It affects up to 20 percent of new mothers, and is in fact considered the most common complication of childbirth. You've probably heard of the baby blues, which passes on its own in a matter of weeks—but postpartum depression is different. Your loved one is not making this up, or exaggerating how she feels. Postpartum depression is much more debilitating and can last for a few months, or if left untreated, it can linger for as long as two years.

Given its elusive origin, postpartum depression affects every woman differently and to varying degrees, but there are a common set of symptoms, some of which you've probably noticed in your loved one. They include:

- mood swings
- anxiety
- feelings of sadness or worthlessness
- panic attacks
- excessive crying
- confusion and difficulty concentrating
- irritability and hypersensitivity
- feeling overwhelmed
- feeling inadequate
- anger
- guilt
- sleep problems
- fatigue
- changes in appetite
- feelings of shame
- lack of interest in sex
- loss of interest in activities she used to enjoy
- lack of interest in family and friends
- intrusive thoughts
- physical symptoms like headaches, chest pains, heart palpitations, and hyperventilation

Now for the good news—postpartum depression is a very treatable illness. Most health-care professionals recommend a two-pronged approach to treatment—medication (in the form of antidepressants or antianxiety medications) and professional therapy. It's important to keep in mind that postpartum depression is a *temporary condition*. With support and treatment, your loved one will return to normal soon.

For Partners of Women with PPD

The partners of women with postpartum depression have it especially hard. You bear the brunt of what she's going through. You have to take care of your new baby, your house, and your partner along with your job and any other responsibilities you may have. You're probably having feelings of guilt, frustration, anger, and exhaustion. These kinds of feelings are completely normal and understandable. Since the birth of the baby, your life has changed considerably, and you certainly weren't prepared for your partner to develop PPD. You're carrying a huge burden, and it's easy to become overwhelmed and even depressed in circumstances like these. But there are things you can do to help you and your partner get through this difficult time.

> *"It was a cruel experience, but I have a better appreciation now of what it's like to be a mother."*
> —Sam T.

How to Help Your Partner

Your partner is feeling very isolated and insecure, and is dealing with some combination of the symptoms that we listed above. She may be unable to express her appreciation for your efforts to help her right now, but don't get frustrated, because they *are* making a difference. Below are some specific ways you can help your partner.

Take time off from work. You should arrange to take as much time off from work as you can so that you can be available for your partner. Just your mere presence around the house will make your partner feel better and less isolated. Besides, the reality is that you *do* have to take on extra responsibility around the house, and it'll be easier and less stressful for you if you can take time off from your nine-to-five job.

One way to do this is to use your sick days and vacation days to take a block of time off. Another option is to take an unpaid leave from your company. Some companies even offer paternity leave. If you're not sure if you're entitled to unpaid leave, start by asking your company's human resources department. Under the **Family and Medical Leave Act (FMLA),** many employers are required by federal law to allow their employees (both men and women) twelve weeks of unpaid family leave after the birth or adoption of a child. At the end of your leave, your employer must allow you to return to your job or a similar job with the same salary, benefits, working conditions, and seniority. You can use your unpaid leave in any way you choose during the first year after your child is born. That means you can take it all at once or, as long as your employer agrees, spread it out over your child's first year by taking it in chunks or reducing your normal weekly or daily work schedule. Even if you're not eligible under the FMLA, you may still be eligible for leave under your state's provisions, which are often more generous than the FMLA. (See the Resources section for a list of places to get more information.)

> *"I was able to arrange for Fridays off from work through the FMLA. I took care of the baby most of the day so my wife could sleep, go to the gym, or go out by herself for a while. It made a big difference for both of us."*
> —Chris F.

Listen to her and reassure her. Your partner is dealing with a great many distressing feelings and emotions, and she needs to talk about them. One of the best things you can do for her is to make yourself available to talk with and really listen to what she has to say. Reassure her that you will support her no matter what. She is painfully aware of how difficult her postpartum depression has made things for you, and she may be afraid that you will leave her. Make sure she knows that you love her and are with her for the long haul.

Keep in mind that you don't need to have all the answers— or any of the answers, for that matter—to be a good listener.

When your partner is talking with you about how she's feeling, what she really needs is for you to believe her and be supportive and sympathetic. She doesn't expect you to "fix" things for her. She may tell you that she doesn't believe she will ever get better. This is a function of her illness. Her depression does not allow her to see a bright and happy future. Reassure her in a gentle way that everything will be all right and that things *will* get better. Instead of saying, "Don't be silly. Of course you'll get better," tell her, "I know it seems like this will never end, but your doctor believes that you'll be your old self again soon, and so do I."

Participate in her treatment. It's very important that you support your partner's treatment choices and participate in the process as much as possible. Seeking help for postpartum depression is difficult for many women, so tell your partner how proud you are of her for reaching out for help. Her treatment will most likely involve antidepressants or antianxiety medication, and she will have to weigh the pros and cons of these medications and make decisions about what she wants to try. This can be an especially difficult decision if your partner is breast-feeding, since some PPD medications can be transferred to the baby through breast milk (see chapter 5 for more information on taking medications while breast-feeding). You can be a sounding board by listening to her thoughts about different medications and helping her sort out what she wants to do. Keep in mind, though, that it is entirely up to your partner whether or not she takes medication for her postpartum depression. Some people have strong feelings about this topic, but this is not the time to express them to your partner or try to influence her decision. If she wants your advice, try to be objective with your answers. Remember, what matters is that your partner gets better. Since PPD is in part a brain chemistry problem, medication has proven very successful in treating it. If she's comfortable taking medication, then it's the right decision for her.

"Attending a therapy session with my partner was the best thing I could have done. I got answers to a lot of questions, and I left the session feeling better about the future and more able to support Sara through this."

—Lisa H.

Her treatment will also probably involve therapy. Ask questions about it and show an interest in her progress. Ask if you can attend a session with her. Not only is this a very strong show of support on your part, but it will also give you the opportunity to ask her therapist questions directly and will provide the therapist with valuable information and insight into your partner's condition.

Don't take things personally. Your partner is in a dark place right now, and it may be impossible for her to express appreciation for everything you're doing to help her and keep things running smoothly. She may even lash out at you out of frustration, irritability, and unhappiness. You might feel as though nothing you do or say is right. Try not to take her behavior personally. She may not be capable of showing her gratitude right now, or may not even realize how much you're really doing, but she is registering it on some level and will be able to better appreciate your efforts as she recovers from PPD.

"My wife was so crabby. She would fly off the handle at the drop of a hat. It took me a while to realize that it wasn't me she was so mad at, it was her PPD. Once I understood that, things got better between us, because I was able to head off a lot of fights."

—Ken B.

However, that doesn't mean you should allow your partner to use you as a whipping post. If she snaps at you for no reason, you can calmly and nicely explain to her why you don't believe you deserved to be treated in such a manner. She already feels guilty about how she's behaving, so try not to snap back or yell at her about it.

Be patient. Once you and your partner have figured out that she has postpartum depression and she begins treatment, you may expect that your life together will return to normal quickly. Unfortunately, that's not going to happen. Recovering from postpartum depression is a process, and you can't expect immediate results. Treatments, such as therapy and medication, take time to have an effect on depression symptoms. Some antidepressants can take up to four weeks to start working. Remind yourself and your partner to be patient. Encourage her to continue treatment, and remind her that things will improve as time goes on.

Help her as much as possible. This may sound like a no-brainer (and you're probably already doing this by default), but do everything you can to help her out around the house and with the baby. She is not capable of accomplishing everything she could before she had the baby, even if she is home all day. Relieving her of some of her duties and giving her time to rest will help speed up her recovery. She is probably feeling overwhelmed by her life and her responsibilities right now, and that's a completely normal symptom of postpartum depression. She may also be feeling stressed and upset that the house is a mess and that she just can't keep up with all that needs to be done. It's unrealistic for her or for you to expect that she can keep the house clean, cook dinner every night, or do most of the things she used to be able to do in the first few months after the baby comes. Even a new mother who does not experience postpartum depression could not do this. Reassure your partner that she doesn't have to get everything done. It takes time to learn how to juggle caring for a baby with managing a house and all of life's other responsibilities. Tell her that you are there to help and that she should take things as slowly as she needs to. As she recovers, she will be able to take over her responsibilities again, and the balance between the two of you will return to normal. In the meantime, here are some things you can do to lighten her load:

- do the dishes
- do the laundry
- cook a meal for the family
- straighten up the house (put clothes and toys away, make sure things aren't strewn all over the floor)
- give the baby his nighttime feedings
- bathe the baby
- do the grocery shopping
- take care of the pets (walk the dog every day, keep the food and water bowls full, empty the kitty litter, and so on)

Give her emotional support. You're offering your partner emotional support when you listen to her when she wants to talk, but don't stop there. Reassure her as often as possible that her postpartum depression is temporary and that she will feel better soon. Make an effort to compliment her on progress that she makes or tasks she gets done. Give her positive feedback on all of her accomplishments. Comment on how good she looks when she gets a haircut or gets dressed up. Tell her often that you love her. Tell her what a good mother she is.

Don't expect sex. Most women with postpartum depression have little interest in sex. A lack of libido is part of the disorder. It has nothing to do with you or how attractive you are to her, so don't take her lack of interest in sex personally. She will regain her sex drive as she recovers and begins to feel more like her old self again. It's also important that you don't try to hurry things along with her. In other words, don't pressure her to have sex before she's ready. Instead, reassure her that you understand, that you'll be patient and you won't leave her because she doesn't want to have sex right now. Women with PPD usually have an increased need for nonsexual touching and gestures of comfort, like hugs, massages, and hand-holding. Give this willingly and often, and assure her that you know it will not turn into sex. This will help her relax and really benefit from your touch.

Help her rest and take breaks. Your partner really needs some downtime, so create opportunities for her to take breaks and rest as often as possible. Give her a chance to sit down for at least a few minutes whenever you're around. Even ten minutes off from the baby will help your partner recharge. Another important way to help your partner get back on her feet faster is to coordinate responsibilities so that she can get more sleep. Taking over one or two of the baby's night feedings will allow her to get a good chunk of sleep during the night. Your partner needs at least four hours of good, uninterrupted sleep each night to complete a sleep cycle and restore her biorhythms. This will go a long way toward making her feel better. If doing the night feedings is impossible for you, you could take the baby out for a walk or to the store a few times a week before or after work so that your partner can take a nap.

You should also encourage your partner to take some time for herself. Alone time is precious for her right now, so try to give her as many opportunities as you can. Encourage her to get out of the house and leave the baby home with you. Suggest she take a walk, go to the gym, or have lunch with friends. If she doesn't feel comfortable about leaving the house, propose that she take a nice long bubble bath or go into her bedroom and watch TV for a while and relax.

> *"Every Saturday I stayed with the baby while my wife went to lunch with her friends. I could tell when she got home that that hour out of the house and time with her friends made her feel a lot better."*
>
> —Jason T.

Encourage joint activities. Spending quality time together is beneficial for both you and your partner. It will help you feel close to each other during this difficult time, and it will make it easier for her to ask for (and for you to give her) the support she needs. Get out of the house together, even for an hour or two. Establish a standing date once every two weeks when someone comes over to babysit and the two of you go out. Go to dinner, take a walk, see a movie—just make sure you leave the house for a while. For those times when leaving the house is impossible, you could order takeout from your favorite restaurant and eat together after the baby goes to bed. Or you could rent a movie that you know she wants to see and watch it together while your baby naps. The point is to find ways to spend time together alone so that you can both have a break from the baby and try to enjoy each other for a while.

How to Take Care of Yourself

Being there to care for your partner is important, but so is taking care of your own health and well-being. It's vital that you make taking care of yourself a priority. Letting yourself get run-down or burned-out will render you incapable of supporting your partner and your family to the best of your abilities, and now is the time they need you the most. Here are some ways you can avoid reaching your breaking point:

Use your support system. Just like your partner, you need to have your own social support system in place to be there for you when you need help. A support system usually consists of your friends and family, as well as coworkers, neighbors, and other acquaintances you feel comfortable turning to. These are the people who can come over to babysit when you need a break, run errands for you, drive your partner to her medical appointments, cook meals, pick up some slack for you at work, and generally do whatever you need to relieve some of your stress and make life a little easier. Don't hesitate to call on your support system when you need help with something, big or small. That's what they are there for. (For a more in-depth discussion on social support systems, see chapter 7.)

Take breaks. You need to take some time off from your partner and your baby in order to recharge. Make sure you're taking an adequate number of breaks each day, and find time to do things that you enjoy every so often. Maybe you can't go golfing every weekend now, but there's no reason why you can't go once or twice a month. Some men feel guilty going out to do something fun when their partner is at home feeling miserable. That's a very nice sentiment, but there's no reason for you to feel bad. You deserve to have some fun and get out of the house for a while. It will make you feel better, it will improve your outlook, and in turn you will be a better support for your partner. If you feel uncomfortable leaving your wife and baby alone, ask a family member or a friend to come over while you're gone to keep her company.

Join a support group. There are support groups out there for fathers, and it's a good idea for you to consider joining one, especially if you're a first-time father. You'll meet other men who are trying to get a handle on fatherhood and are dealing with many of the same issues that you are. You'll learn helpful tips on how to care for and interact with your baby, and it'll help you realize that you're not alone in much of what you're going through. Remember, having a baby is a huge life adjustment—not all of what you're going through is caused by your partner's PPD. Some of it is caused by the inevitable upheaval a new baby brings. Support groups can be a big help in this regard.

There are also support groups available for men whose partners have postpartum depression. Check with Postpartum Support International (PSI) to see what kinds of support groups exist in your area. Postpartum Support International is a nonprofit organization dedicated to helping women who are experiencing perinatal mood disorders such as postpartum depression and providing them and their family members with information and referral services. You can call PSI at 800-944-4773 or visit their Web site at www.postpartum.net. Click on the "Support Groups and Area Coordinators" link on the menu and you'll find a list of support groups categorized by state. If there are no resources listed for your area, contact your state's PSI coordinator. She will be able to put you in touch with local resources.

Talk with someone. It's not a good idea for you to try to keep your feelings inside and go it alone. You need to talk with someone about what you're going through and how it's affecting you. Seeing a professional therapist, even for a few sessions, would be very helpful. Or you could talk with a close friend or family member. You may be surprised by how many people you know who have had personal experience with postpartum depression. What you're looking for is someone you trust who will just listen and not be judgmental. Talking about your experience is a way to get some perspective on your situation. Steer clear of anyone who tries to solve your problems or offers unwanted or biased advice.

Eat, sleep, and exercise. Not only is it important to take care of your mental health, but it's also important to take care of your physical health. Make a concerted effort to eat nutritious foods and get as much sleep as you can. You should also be sure to get some exercise. Exercise is a huge stress reliever, and it will help you get rid of some of your tension and anxiety as well as boost your energy. If you belong to a gym, have someone come over to watch the baby with your partner while you take an hour for a workout. Or you could purchase a baby jogger, which would enable you to walk or run with your baby and not have to leave your partner with any child-care responsibilities. There are also baby seat attachments for bicycles if that sounds more appealing to you.

If You Have Older Children

After the birth of a baby, many changes occur in the household. If you have older children, you may have spent some time during your partner's pregnancy preparing them for the arrival of their sibling and for some of the changes they could expect. But sometimes older children get lost in the shuffle when their mom has postpartum depression and you're juggling so much extra responsibility. Older kids may have expected a certain amount of change, but they certainly never expected Mom to be so different. Even kids who are too young to understand what postpartum depression is will sense that something is wrong and know that their mother's behavior is not normal. They'll notice when Mom is crying, or staying in bed more than usual. They'll notice if she's irritable and yells more often, and if she no longer plays with them or takes them to the park. You need to give them a clear and honest explanation about what is happening. Ideally your partner should talk to the children, but often women with PPD don't feel capable of doing so, so it's up to you to tell them what they need to know. Here are some tips on communicating with your kids about postpartum depression:

- When describing the illness to your kids, don't use words like "depression" or "anxiety." They won't understand what you mean. Instead, use more common descriptive words like "sad," "grouchy," "tired," and "worried."
- Reassure them that they did not cause their mom's postpartum depression and that there's nothing they could have done to prevent her condition.
- Tell them that their mom is getting help and will be better soon.

Be sure to give your children extra attention and kindness—they are likely to be missing that from their mom right now. You should also encourage them to get involved in activities with other family members and friends so that their emotional state is not totally dependent upon their mom's mood. It's best to be honest and open with your kids about what's going on and encourage questions and communication about it. Your kids will be much better able to cope with your partner's PPD if they feel like they know what's wrong with Mommy and can talk about it.

For Family and Friends of Women with PPD

The family and friends of a woman with postpartum depression have a critical role to play in her recovery. You are her support system, and she needs to know that she can turn to you and ask for help when she needs it.

Offer your time and help. The best thing you can do for your loved one is offer her your time and help with whatever she needs. Your loved one is in a very dark and vulnerable place right now, and she's not capable of handling many of her normal responsibilities. She's probably having trouble cleaning up the house and doing any real cooking. She could certainly use someone to come over and babysit for her so that she can take a nap or get out of the house for a little while. Offer her your services. Ask her if you can vacuum the living room for her. Tell her you're going to the grocery store and ask if you can pick anything up for her. Offer to drive her to her medical appointments. Do a load of laundry for her. There are many ways you can help out.

Suggest ways to alleviate stress. Your loved one is under a huge amount of stress, so try suggesting ways that she can alleviate some of it. Encourage her to use her support system—remind her that you are all there for her and that she shouldn't hesitate to ask for help. If your loved one has a comfortable income, you could suggest she hire a nanny for a little while, or a housekeeper to come in once a week to help out. If you plan to suggest this, it's a good idea to do some research so that you can present options to your loved one. She may not have the energy or the inclination to do it herself. You could try to cajole her into getting out of the house. Offer to come over and take a walk around the neighborhood with her and the baby. The fresh air and exercise will do her a world of good.

What to Say and Not to Say

Women with postpartum depression are especially sensitive, so here are a few suggestions to keep in mind when you're interacting with your loved one:

Do be encouraging. Keep reminding your loved one that her situation is temporary and that she's making progress. Keep encouraging her to talk to you about how she's feeling and to express what she needs.

Do compliment her. Tell your loved one what a good mother she is, and compliment her each time you notice she accomplishes something she was unable to do before.

Do respect the fact that she is the mother of her child. If you witness your loved one caring for her baby in a way you don't agree with, don't criticize her or try to correct her. The bottom line is that she is the baby's mother, and how she cares for her baby is her choice. It is not your place to undermine her decisions, and doing so will only make her more unsure of herself.

Don't minimize her experience. When talking to people about their difficulties, many of us tend to say things like "I know how you feel" or compare what they are going through with something we went through. It's perfectly fine for you to express sympathy and compassion for what your loved one is going through, but don't try to empathize. Unless you've had PPD, you can't understand how devastating it is. She might end up feeling misunderstood, and she may not want to confide in you anymore.

Don't criticize. As we said above, women with PPD are extremely sensitive, and many already feel like failures in one sense or another. The last thing they need is criticism right now. Compliment your loved one frequently on her mothering abilities, and keep any negative comments to yourself.

Don't tell her to snap out of it. Your loved one can no more snap out of her postpartum depression than can people with diabetes or arthritis. When a loved one has PPD, don't tell her to smile more or just get over it. She doesn't want to have postpartum depression, but she can't simply will herself into wellness.

Don't assume you know more than she does. Don't tell your loved one what to do or how to do it. The better approach is for you to ask how you can help, and to let her know you're there if she has questions or is looking for advice.

Don't compare her baby with other babies. Many women with postpartum depression have symptoms related to their baby, such as overconcern for their health and well-being or disappointment over the baby's gender. Your loved one may be very sensitive to how her baby "measures up" to other babies, so be careful never to draw comparisons.

Don't make hurtful comments based on outdated beliefs. The world is very different now than it was when our mothers and grandmothers were raising their children, and sometimes it's difficult for older generations to accept the realities of today. Refrain from saying things like "It's so sad you have to put your baby in day care," "I didn't go back to work until you were five," or "You have such a beautiful baby and a wonderful husband. What do you have to be depressed about?" None of these comments are applicable to your loved one's situation, and they will only serve to make her feel worse.

ELEVEN

Your Recovery
and the Future

BY THIS POINT, we hope you have gone to
your health-care practitioner for help with your postpartum depression, have settled on a treatment plan, and have begun to implement
that plan. We also hope you try some of the suggestions you've read
in this book—many of them can help you speed up your recovery. If
you're still thinking about whether you should reach out for help,
consider this: it will take far longer for you to recover from PPD on
your own, without professional help, and you have a much greater
chance of developing it again with subsequent births. Why suffer any
longer than you absolutely have to?

Now that you're on the road to recovery, you're probably won-
dering how long it will take before you feel like your old self again.
Unfortunately, that's impossible to say. The process of recovering
from postpartum depression is different for everyone. But rest assured
that you *will* recover. Most women experience similar stages of recovery, which we describe below, and you can use that information to
gauge where you are in your own recovery. Another good tool for
judging the progress of your recovery is using a scale of one to ten.

One means you are feeling perfect, and ten means you're feeling the worst you've ever felt. Assess how you feel every few weeks, and assign your overall feeling a corresponding number from the scale. You'll see that as your treatment takes effect and you work through your issues, the numbers will get lower and lower. It's important to say that you should never compare your recovery with anyone else's. No two recoveries are the same, and just because someone is recovering faster or slower than you doesn't mean something is wrong.

The First Stage of Recovery

The first stage of recovery begins when you start your treatment. Some women do feel a bit of immediate improvement, but it often takes a few weeks before your medication takes effect or your therapy begins to bring results, so you won't necessarily feel better right away. Having postpartum depression is often likened to being on a roller-coaster ride, because your emotions are unpredictable and can change in the blink of an eye. You'll still be on the roller-coaster ride during the first stage of your recovery, but the ride won't be as rough. Your symptoms will ebb and flow, you will have glimmers of clarity and lucidity, and life will start getting easier.

Often it's the people around you who notice the first signs of improvement. A friend might tell you that you look better or seem happier. Even if you haven't registered this change, these types of comments are usually a sign that treatment is starting to work.

During this first stage, you'll begin to refocus your attention from yourself to others. Postpartum depression causes you to become completely absorbed in what you are going through. Now you'll be able to take an interest in your friends and family again. You'll no longer be constantly dwelling on how bad you feel.

You will also begin to rediscover the activities that used to make you happy and enjoy them once again. You'll want to call your friends on the phone again, go shopping, or go to the beach. This is the first concrete sign of improvement for many women, because resuming old activities makes them feel like their old selves again. It gives them hope for the future, and they begin to truly believe that they will get well.

The Second Stage of Recovery—Remission

The remission stage of recovery is marked by a fluctuation of moods, or lots of ups and downs. This stage is also known as the PMS stage, because your symptoms may take on a cyclical pattern in accordance with your menstrual period. On some days, you'll feel better than you have in a long time. On others, you'll feel like you're right back in the throes of postpartum depression. The PPD is still in control, but you are gaining more and more power and forcing the PPD into remission.

It's important to keep in mind that recovery is a *process,* and you will have both good days and bad days along the way. As your symptoms decrease and the number on the scale of one to ten decreases, you'll have fewer and fewer bad days, but you'll still have some. As you continue to recover, the bad times will become shorter and less intense and the good times will become longer and more pleasurable. Don't let brief moments of feeling like you did before get you down or panic and assume your depression is coming back. Ups and downs are a part of everyday life, and bad days where you feel anxious or blue are normal for everyone. In fact, these blips in your progress mean your treatment plan is working.

This stage is also marked by an increase in energy, so you'll probably start taking on some of the tasks your partner, friends, and family have been helping you with.

The Third Stage of Recovery—Early Recovery

The third stage of recovery, also known as early recovery, is where you begin to pick up the pieces and restore balance in your life. You'll still have some bad days, but the symptoms of your postpartum depression will no longer have the same power over you. The illness is no longer in control of you; you are in control of it. You will have regained much of your confidence, and you'll be able to look back at your postpartum depression and how it affected you. As you continue to recover, you will resume most or all of your normal activities and establish a new schedule for yourself and your family. You will also start thinking about the future. This is actually a significant sign of improvement, because postpartum depression robs most women of their ability to think about or even imagine a future.

A big part of early recovery is learning to accept both the person you have become and your altered perspective on life. Postpartum depression has changed you, and even though you are no longer depressed, PPD has imposed some long-lasting changes on your life. For instance, you may be more susceptible to occasional anxiety or sleep issues. Try to look at these changes as simple limitations that you can live with, not restrictions placed on your life. You know how to deal with these problems now, so they don't need to get in the way of enjoying your life.

As you continue to get better, you may find that some of the people in your support system will continue to worry about you and treat you as though you need more help than you actually do. Be patient with anyone who acts this way—they love you and are simply afraid you may become depressed again. Have a talk with them to gently explain that you're getting better every day and that you're willing and able to handle more responsibility now. Remind them that your health-care practitioners are there to help you monitor how you're feeling, so they don't need to worry about you as much. Hearing this from you will help them treat you more normally.

Fourth Stage—Full Recovery

You have achieved the final stage of recovery when postpartum depression is no longer an issue in your life and you have been weaned from your medications.

Postpartum Depression and Future Pregnancies

As we mentioned earlier, you will reach the point in your recovery where you start to think about the future again. For many women, a big part of the future is deciding whether or not they should expand their family. And if they do decide to try for more kids, will postpartum depression happen to them again?

Unfortunately, if you have postpartum depression once, you have a 50 percent chance of experiencing it again with future pregnancies. The odds increase to over 60 percent if your PPD went untreated. That said, keep in mind that every pregnancy is different—and you are different now, too. You will not necessarily develop postpartum depression again, and if you do, it will likely be less debilitating, because you know what the signs are, you've already developed effective coping mechanisms, and you'll seek help faster. In addition, there are several steps you can take to decrease the likelihood of having a recurrence, or minimize the impact if PPD does happen again.

Make a Plan

It is imperative that you have a treatment plan in place before your next pregnancy so that you can deal with postpartum depression if it occurs again. Go back to the therapist you saw for your first PPD to create this plan. If you didn't see a therapist for your first PPD, make an appointment with one to help you create a plan.

The purpose of this plan is to make as many decisions about your care and response to postpartum depression as you can in advance. This way you can avoid the stress of having to make these decisions after your baby's birth, when you may not be feeling as strong and clearheaded. It will also enable you to get the necessary treatment faster, so you can recover faster.

Make sure your health-care practitioners are well aware that you had PPD before so that they can be on the lookout for symptoms during your pregnancy and be there to help you if it recurs. Your health-care practitioners see many patients, so don't assume they remember your previous postpartum depression. Remind them of your situation, and if you've changed health-care practitioners, make sure to give your new one a detailed account of your experience.

You should also be sure to talk with your health-care practitioners in advance about your medication options. Some women decide to begin medication late in their pregnancy or right after delivery as a preventive measure. Others wait until they begin experiencing symptoms before taking medication. If you used medication to recover from your previous PPD, you know which medications work for you, so there will be no trial-and-error period this time. Your health-care practitioner will immediately prescribe the medication you used during your first bout of PPD, and you will get relief faster.

You may also want to decide whether you're going to breast-feed if you need to be on medication for PPD. As you may recall from chapter 5, antidepressants and other medications used to treat PPD are excreted in breast milk. Although studies show that breast-feeding while on medication poses little risk to your baby, the fact remains that your baby is being exposed to whatever drug you are taking. Whether or not to take medication is a particularly stressful decision for many women, and it can give you great peace of mind to make this decision in advance. There's always room to change your mind if you find yourself questioning your decision when the time comes to take action. (See page 101 in chapter 5 for more information on taking medication while breast-feeding.)

You should also get your partner on board with your treatment plan. Involve him in your decision-making process, and ask him to be on the lookout for any symptoms of depression during your pregnancy and in the first months after you give birth.

Consider the Timing of Your Next Pregnancy

Some experts believe that women who have experienced postpartum depression should wait until their child is three to four years old before having another baby. This way the demands on you may be less severe, because your older child may be more independent and you can focus more easily on caring for your newborn. Older kids can occupy themselves for longer periods of time and can be dropped off for play dates more easily. Your older child may also be better able to handle another episode of postpartum depression if it occurs.

While there's certainly merit to this argument, many women who have experienced PPD choose not to wait so long and experience no adverse effects. Many women prefer to have their children closer together so that they can get through the infant/toddler years faster.

Age may be a factor for you and partner. Some women are in their thirties—even their forties—when they start their families, which can make waiting a long period of time between children unfeasible.

You should also consider if the people in your support system will be available during your postpartum period. For instance, Nancy V. is married to a tax attorney who works extremely long hours from January to April 15. She wisely decided that having a baby during this time period would be too stressful for her.

When thinking about the timing of having another baby, you need to weigh the pros and cons and do what feels right to you. There is no scientific evidence that shows waiting longer between children will decrease your chances of getting postpartum depression again. It's more an issue of how stressful having two young children may be and how that would impact your emotional state.

Get Your Support System in Place

Now that you've been through postpartum depression once, you have identified the members of your social support system and how each person can best help you through a recurrence. Talk with each person and explain that there is a chance you may develop postpartum depression again, so you want to be as prepared as possible. Tell them you already have a treatment plan in place in case it recurs, so this time the PPD should be less debilitating and you will get better more quickly. Explain that regardless of whether you develop postpartum depression again, you'll need their help to get through the first few months with the new baby. This way your support system will be prepared to help you as soon as your baby arrives.

If you did not have the support you needed or wanted after your last pregnancy, now is the time to build that support. If your family and friends weren't aware you had PPD after your last pregnancy, explain to them what it is and how it affected you. Ask them if you can call upon them for help when the baby arrives. You could also try to strengthen your support system by renewing old friendships or joining a women's group. You could meet other women who are expecting through prenatal exercise or education classes.

When you get home from the hospital, don't wait until you hit trouble to call on your support system for help. Contact them immediately so that they can be there to help you take care of the baby as you regain your strength. Have a different friend or family member come over each day for an hour so that you can take a nap or a rest. When you're feeling stronger, use some of that time to leave the house. Take a walk around the neighborhood or go get your nails done.

Be Aware of Your Risk Factors

It is very important that you are aware of your risk factors and do what you can to minimize them before your baby arrives. Some of your risk factors may be unchangeable, such as having a history of childhood abuse, having premenstrual dysphoric disorder, and, of course, a previous postpartum depression. But others, such as marital problems or a weak support system, can be improved.

It's also important to note that you may have some different risk factors with this pregnancy. For instance, perhaps you or your partner have just been laid off, or you have to have an emergency C-section or experience some other kind of traumatic birth experience this time. There are many situations that can make you vulnerable to postpartum depression that you may not have considered with your previous pregnancy, because they didn't apply to you at the time. Be sure to go back and reread chapter 3 to refresh your memory on all the different risk factors for PPD. Once you've assessed your risk factors for this pregnancy, make improvements wherever you can.

Reduce Your Stress

During your pregnancy and your postpartum period, do what you can to lessen the stress in your life. Now is not the time to move into a new home (unless you really have to) or to remodel your current one. If you're working, don't change jobs, overextend yourself, or take on additional responsibilities. That goes for your partner, too, since his stress level has a direct effect on you. After the baby arrives, take as much time off work as you can. Have your partner arrange to do the same. Many women have to go back to work six or eight weeks after they give birth. If this is the case for you, consider talking with your boss about the possibility of working part-time for a few weeks, or even splitting your time between telecommuting and working in the office. Technology has made it easier than ever to work from home, and you may be surprised by how flexible your boss will be. Sue was able to work out a schedule where she worked four days a week—three full days in the office and two half days working from home. It was a great balance for her.

You should also consult your calendar and reschedule any commitments you may have until at least three months postpartum (preferably six months). Your goal is to organize your life so that you'll have less stress, especially during your first few months postpartum.

Divvy Up Responsibilities Before Baby Arrives

Sketch out a plan with your partner in which you divide up the child-care and household responsibilities during your postpartum period. Your partner will need to take on extra duties for a while, and it will be helpful to both of you to figure out what must be done and to know what to expect from each other. Remember, you won't be able to accomplish everything you could before the baby, so don't place that expectation on yourself or your partner. Make a list of tasks that need to be done every day as well as those that can wait a few days or even until you're feeling better. Make a schedule that shows who will take your older children to school or to day care in the morning, who will make dinner, who will have laundry duty, and who will feed the baby during the night for each day of the week. Don't forget to recruit help from your support system and add them to your schedule. This way everyone will be on the same page when the baby arrives. Agree that there will be room for change based on the circumstances you find yourselves in when the time comes.

Work Out Any Relationship Problems

This tip is really part of "Be aware of your risk factors" (see page 202), but it's so important we felt it deserved a section of its own. Trouble in your relationship is one of the biggest contributors to postpartum depression. If you are having problems with your partner, it's crucial that you work them out before the baby arrives. You need to support each other through the postpartum period, especially if you have postpartum depression again, and it will be difficult to do that if you're not getting along. If you find that you've talked but are unable to resolve your differences on your own, we suggest you try going to a relationship counselor. See the Resources section for information on finding a counselor in your area.

Make Labor and Delivery as Stress-Free as Possible

Labor and delivery will be easier for you the second time around, because you've already been through it and will have a greater sense of control over yourself and the situation. Still, there are certain aspects of labor and delivery that will always be out of your control, such as whether you will need a C-section at the final hour or whether your obstetrician will be available to deliver your baby. However, there are some things you can do to ensure a less stressful time for yourself.

It's very important that you have support in the form of your partner or a close friend or family member during your labor and delivery. Make sure that your support person is always reachable so that he or she won't miss being there with you through everything. You might also consider hiring a doula to help you through your upcoming birth. A doula is a trained labor support person who provides you and your partner with emotional and physical support during labor and delivery. Although she is not a medical professional, she can offer a wide range of comfort measures during labor, from massage to aromatherapy to continuous reassurance and coping techniques. Here are some interesting statistics—women supported by a doula during labor have been shown to have:

- 50% reduction in Caesarean rate
- 25% shorter labor
- 60% reduction in epidural requests
- 30% reduction in analgesia use
- 40% reduction in forceps delivery

A doula can help you have the birth experience that you want. She is your advocate and is there to make your childbirth experience easier and less stressful for you. See the Resources section for information on how to find a doula in your area.

You should also pack whatever you need to be comfortable and relaxed at the hospital. Bring your pillow from home or your favorite slippers. If you have an iPod or a Walkman, create a playlist of soothing tunes to listen to during labor.

Make Time for Yourself Every Day

Making yourself a priority and having time to yourself each day was a big part of your recovery from postpartum depression with your previous birth. Don't stop this healthy habit now. Make sure to allot time every day for doing something that makes you feel good. Take a walk, soak in the bath, read a magazine, watch your favorite TV show—it doesn't matter what you do as long as it's for *you*. It's especially important that you continue this practice after you get home with your new baby. That is when you'll need time alone to recharge the most. Many new moms initially find it difficult to fit in time for themselves, and some feel guilty about doing it, but don't let that stop you. You're taking care of yourself, which will make you better able to take care of your family. Everyone benefits.

Make All of Your Preparations Well in Advance

If you need to paint the new baby's room, put up wallpaper, or buy furniture, don't wait until the last minute. Running around in your eighth or ninth month of pregnancy trying to get everything done will cause your stress level to rise sharply. Pack your hospital suitcase a month ahead of time. Buy a gift for your older child from the new baby and vice versa way in advance. Start your preparations early so that you can finish them early and take your time.

Exercise and Eat Right

We highly recommend that you exercise through your pregnancy and your postpartum period. Exercise does so many great things for you. It naturally improves your mood and gives you a feeling of well-being. It will help you keep your weight gain during pregnancy within the normal range. It will boost your self-esteem, and it will improve your cardiovascular health. All of these benefits will make you less susceptible to postpartum depression after your next birth.

Eating healthfully is also important. Your diet is intricately tied to how you feel. Eating poorly or overindulging in junk food can lower your self-esteem, because you know you shouldn't be eating in such an unhealthy way but you're doing it regardless. Make sure you eat a variety of whole grains, plenty of fruits and vegetables, and lean meats and fish. Avoid caffeine, alcohol, and sugar.

Current Research

Since the possibility of developing postpartum depression again with future births is very real, it's to your benefit to keep abreast of new medical developments on the condition. There is still so much we don't know about PPD, and the only way to learn what we need to know is through high-quality scientific research. Research on postpartum depression has been slow-going since it started in earnest in the 1950s, but the medical community's interest in the condition has continued to grow, and some exciting studies are being conducted that will help all of us better understand the condition and improve our ability to treat it more effectively. Knowing the latest research will prepare you to make the most informed decisions you can in case you find yourself struggling with PPD again.

The National Institute of Mental Health (NIMH) sponsors the vast majority of the research studies being done on postpartum depression. The NIMH is one of twenty-seven components of the National Institutes of Health (NIH), the federal government's principal biomedical and behavioral research agency. The NIMH's mission is to conduct research on mental disorders and the underlying basic science of brain and behavior. The institute supports research on these topics at universities and hospitals around the United States. They support the training of more than one thousand scientists to carry out basic and clinical research, and they communicate information to scientists, the public, the news media, and primary care and mental health professionals about mental illnesses, the brain, behavior, mental health, and opportunities and advances in research in these areas. Below we briefly describe some of the studies they are currently conducting.

Effectiveness of Supplemental Calcium in Preventing Postpartum Depression: This study will evaluate the effectiveness of taking supplemental calcium while pregnant in reducing the risk of postpartum depression.

Clinical Trial of Estrogen for Postpartum Depression: Estradiol therapy has a prophylactic effect in women who are at high risk for developing PPD. Preventing a decline in estradiol levels may prevent the onset of PPD. Studies also suggest that estradiol has antidepressant effects in women and may provide a safe and effective alternative to traditional antidepressants in women with PPD. Therefore, this study will evaluate the effectiveness of the female sex hormone 17 beta-estradiol in treating women with postpartum depression.

Group Therapy for Postpartum Depression: This study will compare standard individual treatment with group therapy for the treatment of postpartum depression.

Identification and Therapy of Postpartum Depression: This study will evaluate the effectiveness of a telephone-based depression screening and care management program in treating depression in postpartum women.

Sertraline for the Prevention of Recurrent Postpartum Depression: This study will determine the effectiveness of taking sertraline (better known as the antidepressant Zoloft) within twenty-four hours of giving birth in preventing a recurrence of postpartum depression.

The NIMH may be conducting the most studies on postpartum depression, but they are by no means the only organization interested in furthering our knowledge of the condition. The Chinese University of Hong Kong is conducting a study on the effectiveness of screening for postpartum depression. They are comparing the mental health outcome (at six months postpartum) of mothers who were screened using the Edinburgh Postnatal Depression Scale with those who were not screened.

The Canadian Research Institute for Social Policy is conducting a study to examine the impact of a social support system for mothers affected by postpartum depression and for their infants.

The National Institute of Child Health and Human Development, another branch of the NIH, is doing a study on the differences among depressed mothers' behaviors and how these behaviors influence their infants' reactions. The study also examines how mother-child interactions relate to children's temperament, cognitive (thought-processing) abilities, and other areas of development.

The Brown Center for the Study of Children at Risk at Brown University is conducting a study to examine the effects of maternal antidepressant use and maternal depression on fetal and newborn neurobehavioral development.

The University of Rochester and Forest Laboratories, Inc. in New York are carrying out a study to determine if escitalopram (better known as Lexapro) is effective in the treatment of postpartum depression.

St. Joseph's Healthcare–Hamilton, McMaster University Medical Centre, Joseph Brant Hospital (Brantford), and Women's College

Hospital in Ontario, Canada, are conducting a research study to investigate whether reducing sleep deprivation in new mothers can prevent the occurrence of postpartum depression.

Clearly, progress is being made to further our understanding of postpartum depression. The medical community and the public are finally starting to take postpartum depression seriously and thus validating the struggle that so many women go through after childbirth. We are hopeful that soon we will know why women develop this condition and how we can prevent it. The future looks bright.

A FINAL WORD

POSTPARTUM DEPRESSION IS a harsh illness, because it assaults your body, mind, and spirit. It puts an end to your dreams of what motherhood would be like and marks the beginning of your struggle to let go of impossible expectations, adapt to change, accept the illness, and accept yourself for who you are. Being a mom is hard work, full of challenges and tough times as well as rewards and happiness. The key is to understand that you are human, that you will make mistakes, that you will have both good times and bad, and love yourself regardless.

When you're in the thick of postpartum depression, it's impossible to believe that any good could come of having it. There are no tried-and-true programs for overcoming postpartum depression—every woman's PPD is unique to her, and therefore her treatment and recovery will be unique to her as well. What we've tried to do in this book is give you some guidelines to help you emerge from the darkness of postpartum depression as a better, stronger woman. As two women who have been through postpartum depression ourselves, we can share with you the knowledge that although the journey is difficult, you *will* come through this and be happy again. As with any major life crisis we go through, having postpartum depression is a learning experience that provides us with an opportunity to grow. You will be able to use your experience with PPD as a good frame of reference for other events that will happen in your life. You can be secure in the knowledge that you recovered from postpartum depression, so you can handle anything life throws at you. You will be able to look back and see that your journey of recovery was actually a springboard back into life with a better attitude, a healthy self-love, and the freedom to be yourself.

GLOSSARY

ACTIVATION AFFECT: Term used to describe how your body responds to a chemical when it first enters your system.

AGORAPHOBIA: Anxiety about being in places or situations from which escape might be difficult (or embarrassing) or in which help may not be available if you have a panic attack or panic-like symptoms.

ANTEPARTUM DEPRESSION: Depression that occurs during pregnancy.

ANTIANXIETY MEDICATIONS: (Also see **anxiolytics**) Antianxiety medications are a class of medication used to treat anxiety disorders and anxiety that occurs with depression.

ANTIDEPRESSANTS: Antidepressants are medicines used to help people who have depression. They work by slowing the removal of certain neurotransmitters in the brain, therefore making them more available to the brain.

ANXIOLYTICS: (also see **antianxiety medications**) A class of medication prescribed to treat the symptoms of anxiety.

ATYPICAL ANTIDEPRESSANTS: Atypical antidepressants are a subclass of antidepressants that are chemically unrelated to other antidepressants. They are typically tried when other antidepressants are not effective or have problematic side effects.

BENZODIAZEPINES: (also see **minor tranquilizers**) A class of drugs with sedative, hypnotic, anxiolytic, anticonvulsant, amnestic, and muscle-relaxant properties. They are often used for short-term relief of severe, disabling anxiety or insomnia.

BIPOLAR DISORDER: Also known as *manic-depressive illness,* bipolar disorder is a serious medical illness that causes shifts in a person's mood, energy, and ability to function. Different from the normal ups and downs that everyone goes through, the symptoms of bipolar disorder are severe.

CARBAMAZEPINES: A class of medication that controls seizures and relieves certain types of pain.

DOPAMINE: Dopamine is a type of neurotransmitter that affects the brain processes that control movement, emotional response, and the capacity to feel pleasure and pain.

DOULA: A doula is a trained labor support person who provides emotional and physical support to a laboring woman and her partner.

ENDORPHINS: Opium-like substances produced naturally in the brain that give a feeling of well-being. Production of endorphins is stimulated by many natural circumstances, and also by profound exercise.

ENKEPHALINS: Naturally occurring molecules in the brain that attach to special receptors in your brain and spinal cord to stop pain messages. They also affect other functions within the brain and nervous system.

ESTROGEN: The female sex hormone produced by the ovaries, responsible for the development of female sex characteristics. Estrogen is largely responsible for stimulating the uterine lining to thicken during the first half of the menstrual cycle in preparation for ovulation and possible pregnancy.

FAMILY AND MEDICAL LEAVE ACT (FMLA): Enacted in 1993, the FMLA enables eligible employees to take up to twelve weeks of unpaid leave to meet family needs.

GABA: A chemical messenger in the brain, spinal cord, heart, lungs, and kidneys that sends messages telling the body to slow down. GABA is the primary inhibitory neurotransmitter in the brain.

INTERRUPTED PREGNANCY: A pregnancy that is terminated upon discovering that the fetus suffers from genetic problems, such as trisomy 18.

INTRUSIVE THOUGHTS: Bizarre thoughts about unhappy or violent situations or ideas that you recognize are not normal or realistic.

METOCLOPRAMIDES: A class of antinausea medication that is prescribed for pregnant women.

MINOR TRANQUILIZERS: (also see **benzodiazepines**) A class of drugs with sedative, hypnotic, anxiolytic, anticonvulsant, amnestic, and muscle-relaxant properties. They are often used for short-term relief of severe, disabling anxiety or insomnia.

MONOAMINE OXIDASE INHIBITORS (MAOIs): A class of medication that relieves depression by preventing the enzyme monoamine oxidase from metabolizing the neurotransmitters norepinephrine, serotonin, and dopamine in the brain. As a result, these levels remain high in the brain, boosting mood.

NEUROTRANSMITTER: A chemical that transmits signals between the nerve cells and the brain.

NORADRENERGIC SYSTEM: A system of neurons that is responsible for the synthesis, storage, and release of the neurotransmitter norepinephrine.

NOREPINEPHRINE: A neurotransmitter found mainly in areas of the brain that are involved in governing autonomic nervous system activity, especially blood pressure and heart rate.

OBSESSIVE-COMPULSIVE DISORDER (OCD): A condition in which a person becomes consumed with particular thoughts, impulses, or images.

OBSTETRICIAN: A health-care practitioner who specializes in pregnancy, labor, and delivery.

OMEGA-3 FATTY ACIDS: Also known as alpha-linolenic acid, omega-3s are a fatty acid found in fish and vegetable oils. Omega-3s help prevent the formation of blood clots and reduce the risk of coronary heart disease.

ORALLY BIOAVAILABLE: Term used to describe a medication that is unable to be administered orally.

ORTHOSTATIC HYPOTENSION: Dizziness, faintness, or light-headedness that appears only on standing and is caused by low blood pressure.

PERINATAL MOOD DISORDER: Perinatal mood disorders are potentially devastating conditions that affect women during pregnancy and after childbirth.

POSTPARTUM ADJUSTMENT DISORDER (PPAD): A condition where women feel anxiety, self-doubt, tearfulness, fatigue, and many of the symptoms of the baby blues, except it lasts for their first two months postpartum instead of just two weeks.

POSTPARTUM ANXIETY OR AND/PANIC DISORDER: A condition where women experience excessive and often irrational worries and fears about their babies as well as their own actions.

POSTPARTUM MANIA: A condition where women feel "speeded up" and find it difficult to slow down and relax.

POSTPARTUM OBSESSIVE-COMPULSIVE DISORDER (PPOCD): (also see **obsessive-compulsive disorder**) A form of obsessive compulsive disorder experienced by some women shortly after giving birth. Postpartum OCD typically involves frightening thoughts of harming or killing a baby, but such thoughts are not acted upon.

POSTPARTUM POST-TRAUMATIC STRESS DISORDER (PPTSD): (also see **post-traumatic stress disorder**) A form of post-traumatic stress disorder caused by a traumatic birth experience.

POSTPARTUM PSYCHOSIS (PPP): A rare form of psychosis characterized by delusions or hallucinations experienced by some women shortly after giving birth.

POST-TRAUMATIC STRESS DISORDER (PTSD): An anxiety or panic disorder based on a traumatic experience, such as combat, rape, child abuse, witnessing a violent or troubling event, or any serious medical or psychological trauma.

PREMENSTRUAL DYSPHORIC DISORDER (PMDD): PMDD is a severe form of premenstrual syndrome that affects about 3 to 5 percent of menstruating women.

PREMENSTRUAL SYNDROME (PMS): A range of physical and emotional symptoms that some women experience before their monthly periods.

PROGESTERONE: A female steroid hormone secreted by the ovary; it is produced by the placenta in large quantities during pregnancy.

PROLACTIN: A hormone produced by the pituitary gland that stimulates breast development and milk production.

PSYCHOSIS: An illness that prevents people from being able to distinguish between the real world and the imaginary world. Symptoms include hallucinations (seeing or hearing things that aren't really there, or delusions) and irrational thoughts or fears.

REDUCTION: The term used to describe the act of lessening the amount of fertilized embryos in utero.

SCHIZOPHRENIA: A mental illness in which the person suffers from distorted thinking, hallucinations, and a reduced ability to feel normal emotions.

SELECTIVE SEROTONERGIC REUPTAKE INHIBITORS (SSRIs): SSRIs relieve symptoms of depression by blocking the reabsorption (reuptake) of serotonin by certain nerve cells in the brain. This leaves more serotonin available, which enhances neurotransmission and improves mood. SSRIs are called selective because they seem to affect only serotonin, not other neurotransmitters.

SEROTENERGIC SYSTEM: A system of neurons that is responsible for the synthesis, storage, and release of the neurotransmitter serotonin.

SEROTONIN: A chemical messenger in the brain that affects emotions, behavior, and thought.

TRICYCLICS (TCAs): TCAs work by beefing up the brain's supply of norepinephrine and serotonin levels—chemicals that are abnormally low in depressed patients. This allows the flow of nerve impulses to return to normal.

TYRAMINE: Tyramine is an amino acid normally found in your body that helps regulate blood pressure. It's also found in certain foods. A side effect of monoamine oxidase inhibitors (MAOIs) is that tyramine isn't broken down by the body. High levels of tyramine can cause a marked increase in blood pressure, which may lead to stroke.

URINARY RETENTION: The inability to empty your bladder completely, or at all, despite an urge to urinate.

RESOURCES

POSTPARTUM DEPRESSION

The following resources specialize in PPD or maternal mental health and are the best places to start looking for help and information:

Central New Jersey Maternal and Child Health Consortium
2 King Arthur Court, Suite B
North Brunswick, NJ 08902
Phone: 732-937-5437
Fax: 732-937-5540
www.cnjmchc.org

Health Resources and Services Administration
Maternal and Child Health Bureau
Parklawn Building, Room 18-05
5600 Fishers Lane, Rockville, MD 20857
Hotline: 800-311-BABY (800-311-2229). Hotline number helps pregnant
    women and mothers with newborns identify free or low-cost services for
    themselves and their infants in their communities.

Postpartum Education for Parents
PO Box 6154
Santa Barbara, CA 93160
www.sbpep.org

Postpartum Resource Center of New York, Inc.
109 Udall Road
West Islip, NY 11795
Phone: (631) 422-2255
www.postpartumny.org

Postpartum Support International
927 North Kellogg Avenue
Santa Barbara, CA 93111
Phone: 805-967-7636
Fax: 805-967-0608
www.postpartum.net

We wanted to note that shortly before this book's publication, the non-profit organization Depression After Delivery (D.A.D.), merged with Postpartum Support International and is no longer a separate organization. You can access D.A.D.'s archived Web site at www.depressionafterdelivery.com—they still have some very helpful information and links, but the information has not been updated for at least one year.

Postpartum Stress Center
1062 Lancaster Avenue
Rosemont Plaza, Suite 2
Rosemont, PA 19010
Phone: 610-525-7527
www.postpartumstress.com

POSTPARTUM DEPRESSION AND FATHERS

Postpartum Dads
https://home.comcast.net/%7eddklinker/mysite2/
    Frames_Page.htm

GENERAL SUPPORT FOR FATHERS

Dads Adventure
230 Commerce, Suite 210
Irvine, CA 92602
Phone: 714-838-9670
Toll-free: 800-318-3803
www.newdads.com

Dads Adventure sponsors Boot Camp for New Dads workshops across the country. You can write to the above address for more information or visit their Web site www.bcnd.org.

The National Center for Fathering
P.O. Box 413888
Kansas City, MO 64141
Toll Free: 800-593-DADS
Phone: 913-384-4661
www.fathers.com

WOMEN'S HEALTH

The following resources offer information on general women's health topics as well as postpartum depression and other perinatal mood disorders:

National Women's Health Information Center (NWHIC)
Toll-free: 800-994-WOMAN (800-994-9662)
Toll-free TDD: 888-220-5446
www.4woman.gov

Office on Women's Health (OWH)
U.S. Department of Health and Human Services
200 Independence Avenue, SW, Room 730B
Washington, DC 20201
Phone: 202-690-7650
Fax: 202-690-7172
www.4woman.gov/owh/about/index.htm

American College of Obstetricians and Gynecologists (ACOG)
409 12th Street, SW
Washington, DC 20024-2188
Phone: 202-484-3321
Fax: 202-479-6826
www.acog.com

American Academy of Family Physicians (AAFP)
11400 Tomahawk Creek Parkway
Leawood, KS 66211-2672
Phone: 913-906-6000
www.aafp.org

PMS Research Foundation
PO Box 14575
Las Vegas, NV 89114
Phone: 702-369-9248

Women's Health America
1289 Deming Way
Madison, WI 53717
www.womenshealth.com

DEPRESSION

The following resources are dedicated to major depression but offer good information on postpartum depression as well:

American Psychiatric Association
1400 K Street, NW
Washington, DC 20005
Phone: 202-682-6000
www.psych.org

American Psychological Association (APA)
750 First Street, NE
Washington, DC 20002-4242
Phone 202-336-5500
Toll-free: 800-374-2721
www.apa.org

Depression and Bipolar Support Alliance
730 N. Franklin, Suite 501
Chicago, IL 60601-7204
Toll-free: 800-826-3632
www.dbsalliance.org

International Foundation for Research and Education on Depression
    (iFred)
2017-D Renard Ct.
Annapolis, MD 21401
Phone: 410-268-0044
Fax: 443-782-0739
www.depression.org

National Alliance on Mental Illness
Colonial Place Three
2107 Wilson Blvd., Suite 300
Arlington, VA 22201-3042
Toll-free: 800-950-NAMI (6264)
www.nami.org

NARSAD: The Mental Health Research Association
60 Cutter Mill Rd., Suite 404
Great Neck, NY 11021
Toll-free: 800-829-8289
www.narsad.org

National Council for Community Behavioral Healthcare
12300 Twinbrook Parkway, Suite 320
Rockville, MD 20852
Phone: 301-984-6200
www.nccbh.org

National Institute of Mental Health
NIMH Public Inquiries
6001 Executive Boulevard, Room 8184, MSC 9663
Bethesda, MD 20892-9663
Phone: 301-443-4513
Toll-free: 866-615-6464
www.nimh.nih.gov

National Mental Health Association
1021 Prince Street
Alexandria, VA 22314-2971
Toll-free: 800-969-NMHA (6642)
www.nmha.org

National Mental Health Information Center
P.O. Box 42557
Washington, DC 20015
Toll-free: 800-789-2647
www.mentalhealth.org

Substance Abuse and Mental Health Services Administration (SAMHSA)
U.S. Department of Health and Human Services
5600 Fishers Lane
Rockville, MD 20857
Phone: 301-443-8956
www.samhsa.gov

Substance Abuse and Mental Health Data Archive
The University of Michigan
PO Box 1248
Ann Arbor, MI 48106-1248
Toll-free: 888-741-7242
www.icpsr.umich.edu/SAMHDA

ANXIETY DISORDERS

These sites provide valuable information and resources for those with anxiety issues:

Anxiety Disorders Association of America (ADAA)
11900 Parklawn Dr., Suite 100
Rockville, MD 20852
Phone: 301-231-9350
www.adaa.org

National Institute of Mental Health
6001 Executive Boulevard, Room 8184, MSC 9663
Bethesda, MD 20892-9663
Phone: 301-443-4513
Toll-free: 866-615-6464
www.nimh.nih.gov/healthinformation/anxietymenu.cfm

Children's Mental Health Resources
American Academy of Child and Adolescent Psychiatry
3615 Wisconsin Ave., NW
Washington, DC 20016-3007
Phone: 202-966-7300
www.aacap.org

American Society for Adolescent Psychiatry
PO Box 570218
Dallas, TX 75357-0218
Phone: 972-686-6166
www.adolpsych.org

Research and Training Center on Family Support and
    Children's Mental Health
PO Box 751
Portland, OR 97207-0751
Toll-free: 888-244-0144
Email: rtcpubs@pdx.edu
www.rtc.pdx.edu

EATING DISORDERS

National Eating Disorders Association
603 Stewart St., Suite 803
Seattle, WA 98101
Phone: 206-382-3587
Toll-free Helpline: 800-931-2237
www.edap.org

National Association of Anorexia Nervosa and
    Associated Disorders (ANAD)
PO Box 7
Highland Park, IL 60035
Phone: 847-831-3438
www.anad.org

FOR MORE INFORMATION ON THE FMLA AND FAMILY LEAVE POLICIES, CONTACT:

U.S. Department of Labor
Wage and Hour Division
200 Constitution Avenue, NW
Washington, DC 20210
Phone: 866-487-9243

National Partnership for Women & Families
1875 Connecticut Avenue, NW, Suite 710
Washington, DC 20009
Phone: 202-986-2600
Fax: 202-986-2539
www.nationalpartnership.org

Families and Work Institute
267 Fifth Ave., 2nd Floor
New York, NY 10016
Telephone: 212-465-2044
Fax: 212-465-8637
www.familiesandwork.org

MARRIAGE COUNSELING

The Family and Marriage Counseling Directory
http://family-marriage-counseling.com/index.htm
They offer a directory of professionals by state as well as tips on choosing
    a counselor.

DOULAS

DONA International
PO Box 626
Jasper, IN 47547
Toll-free: 888-788-DONA (3662)
Fax: 812-634-1491
www.dona.org

Doula Network
www.doulanetwork.com

Birthpartners.com
National Childbirth Providers Directory
www.birthpartners.com

Doulaworld.com
www.doulaworld.com/doula/cfml/main/index.cfm

SUGGESTED READING

Beck, Cheryl Tantano and Jeanne Watson Driscoll. *Postpartum Mood and Anxiety Disorders: A Clinician's Guide.* Boston, MA: Jones and Bartlett, 2006.

Bennett, Shoshana, PhD, and Pec Indman, EdD, MFT. *Beyond the Blues: A Guide to Understanding and Treating Prenatal and Postpartum Depression.* San Jose, CA: Mood Swings Press, 2003.

Blumfield, Wendy. *Life After Birth: Every Woman's Guide to the First Year of Motherhood.* Rockport, MA: Element Books, 1992.

Briggs, Gerald. *Drugs in Pregnancy and Lactation: A Reference Guide to Fetal and Neonatal Risk.* Philadelphia: Lippincott Williams & Wilkins, 2005.

Casey, Karen. *Each Day a New Beginning: Daily Meditations for Women.* Center City, MN: Hazelden Books, 1996.

Chevalier, A. J. *Shudda, Cudda, Wudda: Affirmations to Cope With Self-Doubt.* Deerfield Beach, FL: Health Communications, 1996.

Dean, Amy E. *Night Light: A Book of Nighttime Meditations.* Center City, MN: Hazelden Books, 1996.

Dunnewold, Ann, PhD, and Diane G. Sanford, PhD, *Postpartum Survival Guide.* Oakland, CA: New Harbinger, 1994.

Groves, Dawn. *Meditation for Busy People: 60 Seconds to Serenity.* Novato, CA: New World Library, 1993.

Hale, Thomas. *Medications and Mothers' Milk (12 ed.).* Amarillo, TX: Hale Publishing, L.P., 2006.

Johnson, Spencer. *One Minute for Yourself.* New York: Quill, 1998.

Kleiman, Karen R. and Valerie D. Raskin. *This Isn't What I Expected: Overcoming Postpartum Depression.* New York: Bantam Books, 1994.

Kleiman, Karen. *What Am I Thinking? Having a Baby After Postpartum Depression.* Philadelphia: Xlibris, 2005.

Louden, Jennifer. *Woman's Comfort Book: A Self-Nurturing Guide for Restoring Balance in Your Life.* San Francisco: HarperCollins, 1992.

Misri, Shaila. *Shouldn't I Be Happy: Emotional Problems of Pregnant and Postpartum Women.* New York: Free Press, 2002.

Peisner, Paula. *Finding Time: Breathing Space for Women Who Do Too Much.* Naperville, IL: Sourcebooks, 2004.

Placksin, Sally. *Mothering the New Mother: Women's Feelings and Needs After Childbirth: A Support and Resource Guide,* 2nd ed. New York: New Market Press, 2000.

Rosenberg, Ronald, MD, et al. *Conquering Postpartum Depression: A Proven Plan for Recovery.* Cambridge, MA: Da Capo Press, 2003.

Saavedra, Beth Wilson. *Meditations for New Mothers.* New York: Workman, 1992.

Sebastian, Linda. *Overcoming Postpartum Depression and Anxiety.* Omaha, NE: Addicus Books, 1998.

Schaef, Anne Wilson. *Meditations for Women Who Do Too Much.* New York: Harper, 1989.

Sichel, Deborah, MD, and Jeanne Watson Driscoll. *Women's Moods: What Every*

Woman Must Know About Hormones, the Brain, and Emotional Health. New York: Harper Paperbacks, 2000.

Vienne, Veronique. *The Art of Doing Nothing: Simple Ways to Make Time for Yourself.* New York: Clarkson Potter, 1998.

Books Specifically for Fathers

Barron, James D. *She's Had a Baby: And I'm Having a Meltdown.* New York: Harper Paperbacks, 1999.

Kleiman, Karen. *The Postpartum Husband: Practical Solutions for Living with Postpartum Depression.* Philadelphia: Xlibris, 2001.

Recommended Web sites

www.babycenter.com
www.emorywomensprogram.org
www.everythingmom.com
www.womensmentalhealth.org
www.storknet.com

Lactation Resources

Lactation Resource Center, Inc.
Toll-free: 800-801-MILK

Le Leche League International
www.lalecheleague.org
If you don't have access to a computer, look in your local telephone directory. Many La Leche League groups have listings in the white pages or Yellow Pages. Some are also listed in the free blue pages for nonprofit organizations, as well. If there is no listing under "La Leche League," look under headings labeled "breast-feeding" or "lactation." In some places La Leche League will be listed under "community resources" or "women's health." You can also call 800-LALECHE (US), or 847-519-7730. The second number provides access to an automated system for finding LLL leaders in the United States by entering a local zip code. In Canada, telephone 800-665-4324, or 514-LALECHE for a French-speaking leader.

International Lactation Consultant Association
http://gotwww.net/ilca
You can plug your zip code into this site and get the names and contact information for lactation consultants in your area.

Medication and Breast-feeding Resources

Breast-feeding Pharmacology
http://neonatal.ttuhsc.edu/lact/index.html
Dr. Thomas Hale is an experienced clinical pharmacologist with many years of lecturing in all areas of pharmacology and therapeutics. He currently is considered a leading expert in the use of medications in breast-feeding women and travels worldwide lecturing on the topic of using medications in breast-feeding mothers. His site has lots of information on breast-feeding and medications, and the information is cutting-edge.

Yoga, Meditation, and Guided Imagery Resources

We've provided only one general resource here, because yoga, meditation, and guided imagery are very personal practices. In order for them to work, you must design your own practice based on your personal needs. You'll most likely need to try out several different styles or programs before you find what works for you, so please don't get discouraged.

Health Journeys
Resources for the Mind, Body and Spirit
www.healthjourneys.com
Toll-Free: 800-800-8661
Belleruth Naparstek's site offers extremely useful information about yoga, meditation, and guided imagery as well as a wide selection of tapes, CDs, and MP3 downloads to choose from.

Self-Help Clearinghouses

For help in finding or forming a mutual help support group for any type of illness, disability, addiction, personal loss, parenting problem, or other stressful life problem, there are local Self-Help Clearinghouses in many parts of the country available to help. They can advise you if there is any self-help group near you to meet your needs. Most clearinghouses can also help if you are interested in joining with others to start a new group by providing suggestions, resource materials, and possibly training workshops or publicity in their newsletter. A search engine to find a Self-Help Clearinghouse near you can be found at www.selfhelpweb.org/links.html. You can also check http://mentalhelp.net/selfhelp.

UNITED STATES

Alabama
    Birmingham 205-251-5912
Arizona
    Statewide 800-352-3792 (in AZ) or 602-231-0868

Arkansas
  Northeast area 501-932-5555
California
  Modesto 209-558-7454; Sacramento 916-368-3100; Davis 916-756-8181; San Diego 619-543-0412; San Francisco 800-273-6222 or 415-772-4357
Connecticut
  Statewide 203-789-7645
Illinois
  Statewide 773-481-8837; Champaign 217-352-0099; Macon 217-429-HELP
Iowa
  Statewide 515-576-5870 or 800-952-4777
Kansas
  Statewide 800-445-0116 (in KS) or 316-978-3843
Massachusetts
  Statewide 413-545-2313
Michigan
  Statewide 517-484-7373 or 800-777-5556 (in MI); Benton Harbor 800-336-0341 (in MI) or 616-925-0594
Missouri
  Kansas City 816-822-7272 (24 hours); St. Louis 314-773-1399
Nebraska
  Statewide 402-476-9668
New Jersey
  Statewide 973-625-7101; TDD 973-625-9053
New York
  Manhattan 212-586-5770; Westchester 914-949-0788, ext. 237; Brooklyn 718-875-1420; Broome 607-771-8888; Cattaragus 716-372-5800; Dutchess 914-473-1500; Erie 716-886-1242; Fulton 518-736-1120; Monroe 716-256-0590; Montgomery 518-842-1900, ext. 286; Niagara 716-433-3780; Oneida 315-735-4463; Onondaga/Syracuse 315-474-7011; Orange/Sullivan 800-832-1200 or 914-294-7411; Rockland 914-639-7400, ext. 22; St. Lawrence 315-265-2422; Saratoga 518-664-8322; Steuben 800-346-2211 (in NY) or 607-936-4144; Tompkins 607-273-9250; Ulster 914-339-9090; Wyoming 716-786-0540; Long Island 516-626-1721 (outside Long Island) or 888-SELF-HELP (on Long Island)
North Carolina
  Mecklenberg 704-331-9500
North Dakota
  Fargo 701-235-SEEK
Ohio
  Dayton 513-225-3004; Toledo 419-475-4449
Oregon

Northwest OR/Southwest WA 503-222-5555
Pennsylvania
Pittsburgh 412-261-5363; Scranton 717-961-1234; Lehigh Valley 610-865-4400
South Carolina
Richland/Lexington 803-791-2800
Tennessee
Knoxville 423-584-9125; Memphis and Shelby 901-323-8485
Texas
Statewide 512-454-3706; Dallas 214-871-2420; Houston 713-522-5161; Tarrant 817-335-5405; San Antonio 210-826-2288
Utah
Salt Lake City 801-978-3333

CANADA

Calgary 403-262-1117
Toronto 416-487-4355
Nova Scotia 902-466-2011
Vancouver 604-876-6086
Prince Edward Island 902-628-1648
Winnipeg 204-589-5500 or 204-633-5955

Source: Joyce Venis, RNC and Penelope Prosperi, LCSW. *A Guide to Starting and Maintaining a Depression After Delivery (DAD) Support Group*

REFERENCES

Chapter 1

www.pregnancy-info.net/postpartum_anxiety_and_panic.html.

Laurence Kruckman and Susan Smith, "An Introduction to Postpartum Illness," www.postpartum.net/in-depth.html.

Kristen Brooks Hope Center [Internet]. Jane I. Honikman, MS, "The Postpartum Scientific Movement," www.hopeline.com/1-1/honikman/default.asp.

C. Neill Epperson, MD, "Postpartum Major Depression: Detection and Treatment," www.aafp.org/afp/990415ap/2247.html.

Laura Flynn McCarthy, "The Truth about Postpartum Depression." *Parents,* Oct. 2001.

Chapter 2

Dunnewold, Ann, PhD, and Diane G. Sanford, PhD, *Postpartum Survival Guide.* Oakland, CA: New Harbinger, 1994.

Chapter 3

Margaret L. Moline, PhD, David A. Kahn, MD, Ruth W. Ross, MA, Lori L. Altschuler, MD, and Lee S. Cohen, MD., "Postpartum Depression: A Guide for Patients and Families," www.psychguides.com/DinW%20postpartum.pdf, March 2001.

"Fussy Babies and Postpartum Depression Linked, Study Finds," www.sciencedaily.com/releases/2006/05/060502090732.htm, May 2, 2006.

C. Neill Epperson, MD, "Postpartum Major Depression: Detection and Treatment," www.aafp.org/afp/990415ap/2247.html.

Wisner K. L., et al. (2002). "Postpartum depression." *New England Journal of Medicine* 347(3): 194–99.

Kathe Gallagher, MSW, "Postpartum Depression," www.peacehealth.org/kbase/topic/major/tn9653/whn2call.htm.

Mary Shomon, "Postpartum Thyroid Problems: Frequently Asked Questions about Thyroid Problems after Pregnancy," www.thyroid-info.com/articles/postpartum.htm.

Ilyene Barsky, LCSW. "Postpartum Depression: Who is at Risk?" www.geocities.com/ppdflorida/risk.htm.

CHAPTER 4

"A Postgraduate Medicine Special Report," March 2001. Margaret L. Moline, PhD, David A. Kahn, MD, Ruth W. Ross, MA, Lori L. Altschuler, MD, and Lee S. Cohen, MD.

R. Kumar and M. K. Robson. "A prospective study of emotional disorders in childbearing women." *British Journal of Psychiatry.* 1984; 144:35–47.

M. W. O'Hara and A. M. Swain. "Rates and risk of postpartum depression—a meta-analysis." *International Review of Psychiatry.* 1996; 8:37–54.

"Edinburgh Postnatal Depression Scale," www.hfs.illinois.gov/mch/edinburgh.html.

Indiana Perinatal Depression Consensus Statement, http://www.indianaperinatal.org/files/education/ppdconsen2005.pdf, April 2005.

"Postpartum Depression," www.mcmanweb.com/article-32.htm

A. M. Llewellyn, Z. N. Stowe, and C. B. Nemeroff. "Depression during pregnancy and the puerperium." *Journal of Clinical Psychiatry.* 1997; 58 (suppl 15): 26–32.

CHAPTER 5

Mayo Clinic staff, "Postpartum depression," http://www.mayoclinic.com/health/postpartum-depression/DS00546, June 9, 2006.

Thomas Hale, PhD, "Using Antidepressants in Breastfeeding Mothers," www.kellymom.com/health/meds/antidepressants-hale10-02.html#Paxil.

Massachusetts General Hospital, Center for Women's Health, "Breastfeeding and Psychiatric Medications," www.womensmentalhealth.org/topics/breastfeeding.html.

TheHealthCenter.info, "Modern Depression Medication Reference," http://www.thehealthcenter.info/adult-depression/depression-medications.htm.

"Complementary Therapies in Treatment of Postpartum Depression" *Journal of Midwifery & Women's Health* 49(2): 96–103, 2004.

HealthyPlace.com, "Psychiatric Medications Pharmacology," www.healthyplace.com/medications/index.asp.

"Side Effects of Medications," National Institute of Health Publication No. 99-3561, www.allaboutdepression.com/med_02.html.

HealthyPlace.com, "Paxil in Late Pregnancy May Cause Problems," http://www.healthyplace.com/Communities/depression/treatment/antidepressants/articles/004.asp, May 7, 2002.

Caron Zlotnick, Ph.D., Sheri L. Johnson, Ph.D., Ivan W. Miller, Ph.D., Teri Pearlstein, M.D. and Margaret Howard, Ph.D., *"Postpartum Depression in Women Receiving Public Assistance: Pilot Study of an Interpersonal-Therapy-Oriented Group Intervention," American Journal of Psychiatry* 158:638-640, April 2001.

National Center for Complementary and Alternative Medicine, "The Use of Complementary and Alternative Medicine in the United States," http://nccam.nih.gov/news/camsurvey_fs1.htm, September 2004.

CHAPTER 7

R. Small, J. Astbury, S. Brown, and J. Lumley. (1994) "Depression after childbirth: Does social context matter?" *Medical Journal of Australia* 161(8): 473–77.

M. O'Hara, L. Rehm, and S. Campbell. (1983) "Postpartum depression: A role for social network and life stress variables." *Journal of Nervous and Mental Disease* 171(6): 336–41.

Nanniesandmore.com, www.nanniesandmore.com/baby-nurses.html.

CHAPTER 8

Kaplan PS, Bachorowski J, Zarlengo-Strouse, P, "Child-directed speech produced by mothers with symptoms of depression fails to promote associative learning in 4-month old infants,"*Child Development* 1999; 70:560–70.

Ngozi Onunaku, MA, "Improving Maternal and Infant Mental Health: Focus on Maternal Depression," http://www.healthychild.ucla.edu/PUBLICATIONS/Maternal%20Depression%20Report%20FINAL.pdf, July 2005.

Florida State University Center for Prevention & Early Intervention Policy, "What is Infant Mental Health?" http://72.14.209.104/search?q=cache:K37gZ2gqXbsJ:www.cpeip.fsu.edu/project.cfm%3FprojectID%3D31+what+is+infant+mental+health&hl=en&gl=us&ct=clnk&cd=10&client=firefox-a.

Harvard Health Publications,"Depression During Pregnancy and After," www.health.harvard.edu/newsweek/Depression_During_Pregnancy_and_After.htm.

Anne D. Walling, "Effects of Postpartum Depression on Children," *American Family Physician,* Nov. 1, 1998.

CHAPTER 11

Doulanetwork.com; Marshall H. Klaus, *Mothering the Mother: How a Doula Can Help You Have a Shorter, Easier and Healthier Birth* (Reading, MA: Addison-Wesley, 1993).

Participating in NIH Research 1, http://clinicalcenter.nih.gov/participate/healthyvolunteers/newsletter_0102.shtml.

www.wrongdiagnosis.com/p/postpartum_depression/intro.htm.

ACKNOWLEDGMENTS

I'**D LIKE TO** thank my husband, Chris Fisher, for being my greatest support and the best friend I could ever hope for. He did more than his fair share of feedings and diaper changes so I could work on this book. I'd also like to thank my son Jack, who made this book possible—it was all worth it to have you. I've got to thank my parents, Ann and Steve McCloskey, and my brother Brian, who encouraged me the whole way through, and my friends Laura Bernann and Wendie Carr, who were there for me through it all.

—SM

I have to thank Malcolm, my husband and soul mate. Without his love, encouragement, support, occasional pushing, understanding, patience, belief in me, and his willingness to share me with so many others, this would not have been a dream come true. Equally important is my son Mark, whose birth started this journey many years ago. Without him, all this would never have been possible. I'd also like to thank everyone who thinks that I've forgotten them. I would never do that. You know who you are and you'll always be with me. I'd like to thank all my wonderful patients and their families for their trust and confidence in me. I am honored to see them turn into the women they were meant to be—themselves. My heartfelt thanks go to Sue McCloskey for asking me to do this labor of love with her and for the courage she has shown by telling her story. I want to thank my mother, Ann, who gave birth to me. She had the ability to make all things better and life worth living. Lastly, I'm grateful to God for giving me the ability to survive so that I could help others even though I was very angry with him during my PPD. I vowed that I would always do all that I could so that women would not have to suffer in silence as I did. Through all my pain I realized that that was God's plan.

We'd both like to thank Matthew Lore, publisher of Marlowe & Company, for believing in us and giving us the opportunity to write this book. Thanks to Vince Kunkemueller for guiding the book through the production process, Jill Hughes for the copyediting, Jesse A. Weissman for the proofreading, and Vivian Ghazarian for the wonderful cover design. We'd also like to thank publicity director Wendie Carr for the fantastic job she did in promoting our book.

INDEX

A

abortion, 62
abuse, 64–65, 166
activation affect, 97, 213
acupuncture, 114
adapting to change, 66
addiction, 62
adoption, 62
advanced practice nurse, 106
age of mother, 71–72
agoraphobia, 17, 31, 213
alcohol, 129
alprazolam (Xanax), 100
alternative medicine, 113–17
amitriptyline (Elavil), 96
Anafranil (clomipramine), 96
anger, 37–38
antepartum depression, 9, 14, 213
anti-mania medications, 100
antianxiety medications, 93, 99–100,
    103, 213
antidepressants, 93–98, 102, 213
antipsychotics, 100
anxiety, 29–30, 59, 222–23
anxiolytics, 99, 213
appetite changes, 43–44, 129–30
Ativan (lorazepam), 100, 103
atypical antidepressants, 94–95, 213
Aventyl (nortriptyline), 96

B

baby
    bonding, 47, 152
    colic, 66–67
    disinterest in, 47–48
    gender, 67
    hypervigilance, 46–47
    PPD effects on, 151–62
    reading to, 159–60
baby blues, 13–15, 79
baby nurse, 144
Beck, Cheryl Tatano, 92
behavioral therapy, 110
Belly Button Book, 160
benzodiazepines, 99–100, 213–14
Berchtold, Nancy, 24
Big Red Barn, The, 160
biofeedback, 114
bipolar disorder, 22, 58, 214
books for children, 160
Boynton, Sandra, 160
breast-feeding
    lactation consultant, 142–43
    and medications, 101–4
    resources, 226–27
    risk of PPD, 55–56
*Brown Bear, Brown Bear, What Do You
    See?*, 160
Brown, Margaret Wise, 159–60